Reclaim
VITALITY

A guide to **exit conventional medicine** and live naturally

Dr. Nick Wilson
& Leah Wilson, JD

Foreword by Joel Salatin

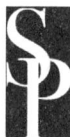

Skyhorse Publishing

Skyhorse Publishing books may be purchased in bulk at special discounts for
sales promotion, corporate gifts, fund-raising, or educational purposes. Special
editions can also be created to specifications. For details, contact the Special Sales
Department, Skyhorse Publishing, 307 Fifth Avenue, 4th Floor, New York,
NY 10016 or info@skyhorsepublishing.com.

Skyhorse® and Skyhorse Publishing® are registered trademarks of Skyhorse
Publishing, Inc.®, a Delaware corporation.

Visit our website at www.skyhorsepublishing.com.
Please follow our publisher Tony Lyons on Instagram @tonylyonsisuncertain.

10 9 8 7 6 5 4 3 2 1

Library of Congress Cataloging-in-Publication Data is available on file.

Hardcover ISBN: 978-1-5107-8593-9
eBook ISBN: 978-1-5107-8594-6

Cover design by Seth Lunsford

Printed in the United States of America

Contents

Foreword

by Joel Salatin

I've been waiting for the breakthrough, breakout book in the wellness field for some time: here it is. You won't find a better philosophical and practical expression of VITALITY than this fabulous book.

What Dr. Nick and Leah Wilson are trying to do in the human context matches perfectly with what I've seen during my farming career. When our family came to this property in 1961, it was the most gullied rockpile of a worn-out place in the whole region. Now sixty-five years later, it's arguably the most productive, abundant landscape in the area.

How did such transformation occur? Essentially, our family, starting with my dad, asked how nature works and then tried to mimic it as closely as possible in commercial production. Animals move; they don't stay cooped up indoors with no exercise or sunshine. This simple notion drives nearly all the innovative portable sheltering, control, and watering systems we use today.

How does nature build soil? Not with 10-10-10 chemical fertilizer, but with decomposing formerly living material. Whether it's manure or decaying plants, carbon is what drives all fertility. And in nature, it doesn't come from far away; it's on sight. Leaves don't blow very far. Animals don't walk too far. Even birds drop manure near where they picked up bugs and seeds. Earthworms hype up minerals and enzymes in the soil through their alimentary canal. Farms are not supposed to be dependent on laboratories and far-off mines.

Today, even though our farm raises thousands and thousands of animals, we literally do not have a vet bill. How can that be? When livestock receives its full complement of nutrition, exercise, and sanitation, in a habitat that allows animals to fully express their distinctiveness (the pig-ness of the pig) they achieve extreme vitality. This principle we see in plants fertilized with good compost and animals enjoying a stress-free, happy life is exactly what the Wilsons, in this fabulous book, bring to the human counterpart.

A handful of times in my life, our farm has experienced a disease outbreak in our livestock. Every single time, it's been my fault. I either deprived them of something essential nutritionally, let them get stressed through crowding or lack of sanitation, or put them in a situation that overran their immune capacity. If we have a sick animal, we don't assume it's pharmaceutically challenged. Our first question is "what did I do to enable a wellness-default position to be overcome?" We don't vaccinate, medicate, or exterminate.

This lifetime observing nature's proclivity toward vitality affirms exactly what this book promotes in every detail. Nature's default position is wellness; if something is sick, it's not because we're suddenly suffering from assaults from nefarious sickness gods. Something is out of whack. It could be structural, like spinal misalignment. It could be spiritual with a vengeful attitude or unforgiveness. It could be because we're clogged with a bunch of unpronounceable junk from ultra processed or chemicalized food. This book drills down on the real causes of maladies and offers real hope and help for all of us to enjoy true vitality.

* * *

Dad was late coming home for chores, so when I finished milking my Guernsey cow, I went ahead and started milking his. We didn't own them separately; he just always milked Crooked Tail, and I milked Gertrude.

He had gone with Mom to get the urologist's report on a prostate biopsy. A couple of months earlier, a routine physical led his regular doc-tor to encourage the biopsy because the prostate seemed a bit enlarged. The barn where I was milking had that irregular light that shines through dusty places before sunset. It wasn't dark but outside was far brighter.

Dad was a power of a man. Strong, vibrant, ex-Navy pilot from World War II, bigger than life. I had returned to the farm full-time a couple of years earlier, in 1982, about the same time he moved his accounting practice home. He was thrilled to see his farming dream, never truly realized, picked up by a son, and I enjoyed his mentorship, sharp pencil, and ability to design and think outside the box. We were a symbiotic pair.

I expected him home anytime. About halfway through finishing milking his cow, a strange man walked through the barn door. I didn't recognize him. It was Dad. I tear up just writing this sentence. My lack of recognition only lasted a second, but I'll never forget that momentary lapse.

"I have the big C," he announced, voice quivering. "Prostate cancer," he added, with the resignation that comes with a death sentence. No appellate court. No jury. Just cancer. He literally died in an afternoon. His countenance drooped in beaten resignation. I didn't know what to say. What could I say? I was in my late twenties, and he was in his early sixties.

The next step was what we call "conventional cut and burn" therapy. Implanted radioactive gold beads, surgery. It took about five years to finally get him; he passed at sixty-six and I was only thirty-one. That's young to lose your dad. I still miss him every day.

Those things affect you. One thing it did to me was make me never want a physical. I've never had one since I went to college at eighteen. I'm now pushing sixty-nine. I'm convinced—perhaps wrongly—that he would have lived much longer had he never gotten that physical. He was in great shape and physically active. We shoveled manure together; threw hay together; loaded firewood together; ran chainsaws together.

I've decided that as long as I feel great and energetic, I don't need someone poking around filling my head with defeat. I've got important things to do. I wake up every day excited to continue a sacred ministry that Dad and I schemed together to build. He didn't completely lose vision. My favorite memento from him is a yellowed piece of paper he wrote on from his sickbed a few months before passing.

He called me into the bedroom: "Bring a pencil and paper." My wife, Teresa, and I were seven years into our Polyface Farm adventure. We lived in the attic of the farmhouse, drove a jalopy, didn't have a TV (still don't), ate out of our garden and from the farm, and were making financial headway. We'd opened a savings account because we finally had some money left over at the end of the year. We could exhale: "We're gonna make it."

What did Dad want to do? He wanted to brainstorm how many salaries could be generated from our little farm. He might have been down, but he wasn't out. We sat together and he wrote out twenty-two salaries. Today we generate twenty-two salaries. And I still have the paper.

I could die tomorrow. I've instructed my family not to resuscitate me for any reason. I don't want to go through debilitating end-of-life entanglement in the medical system. I've run my course, finished the race, and it'll be okay. I don't fear sickness. I don't lie awake wondering how many years I have left.

I'm grateful for every day God lets me represent His desire for our farm and our community. I'm grateful for our team. I've forgiven the folks who ripped us off over the years. I don't resent the folks who call me a bioterrorist, Typhoid Mary, or starvation advocate. I have a mission, a vision, and embrace each day enthusiastically. I drink out of the cow trough to stimulate my microbiome, eat great food from our farm, sweat routinely doing chores, and enjoy long sleepy nights.

I'm known as the one who never gets sick. Is it presumptuous or prideful to make such a statement? I don't think so. It's a result of lots of lifestyle, spiritual, emotional, and physical positive practice.

* * *

In *Reclaim Vitality*, Dr. Nick and Leah coach us through the stories we've been told, the new stories we need to hear, and ultimately how to tell healing stories to ourselves. Phrases like "medical monotheism" penetrate our understanding of what's wrong. Labeling health insurance a "gatekeeper" rather than a safety net is precise truth spoken in an unusually direct manner. Things are too dysfunctional to tiptoe around what is broken.

What if my dad had read this book and looked at his prostate issues as, "I'm just recalibrating?" I think the outcome would have been completely different, but almost nobody in our modern society advocates this kind of narrative.

"Fear isn't just psychological; it's biochemical. Chronic fear floods the body with stress hormones, weakens the immune system, and alters gene expression." How many of us worry about becoming chronically ill? Losing our minds when we get old? The Wilsons explain how and why to rewire our thinking to create protective hedges around our health rather than immunologically compromised breaches.

The last half of the book explains alignment and what we should eat, with checklists to determine where we are on a continuum and then objectives of where we need to go. Ultimately practical on a subject that often mires in subjective nebulous imprecision, this book is like a road map to vitality.

Too often we view wellness as simply not being sick; if we can get our feet out of bed in the morning and dress ourselves, we're fine. But this book dares to move us beyond that mediocrity into a place of true vitality. I don't know about you, but that's exactly where I want to be. If you take the advice in this book, begin practicing it with intention and consistency, your health future will probably be different than that of most of the folks you know.

The time to make changes for the better is today, right now. Knowing what to do begins right now with this great book. Enjoy.

INTRODUCTION

How We Got Here: The Broken System and the Path Forward

The doctor of the future will give no medication but will interest his patients in the care of the human frame, diet, and in the cause and prevention of disease.
                                                              —Thomas Edison

What if everything you need for health, clarity, and energy is already inside you? What if the constant search for solutions—another diet, another doctor, another detox—is actually leading you further away from what you really need? This book isn't about another health trend; it's about returning to the timeless principles that govern health and healing.

For nearly two decades, people have turned to me for health advice. It's been my passion, it's my job, and what I've dedicated my life to mastering. As a doctor and natural health advocate, I help patients and clients transform their lives naturally. But it wasn't always this way. My journey started out with unexplainable recurring suffering and a frustrating search for answers that led me nowhere.

Nick: From Peak Fitness to a Chronic Disease Diagnosis
No one would have known I was falling apart. At eighteen, I looked the part: clear skin, muscular build, 6 percent body fat. I lived in the gym. But inside, my body was spiraling.

The first signs came quietly. A few digestive issues here and there. I

x

ignored them. Until I couldn't. Soon, I was sprinting to the bathroom five, sometimes ten times a day. Blood in the toilet became a regular sight. Something was clearly wrong.

Doctors ran tests, shrugged, and handed me a vague diagnosis: *Inflammatory Bowel Disease.* They gave me prescriptions. Daily meds with no end in sight. I felt there had to be a better way. I just didn't know where to look.

But the damage had already begun long before the diagnosis. Back in high school, I took a medication called Accutane. Like most kids, I trusted the process. A doctor prescribed it for acne, and I followed directions. I didn't overdose. I didn't misuse it. I took what I was told to take.

What no one told me was that Accutane is a synthetic form of vitamin A so potent it's classified as a chemotherapy agent. It can alter liver function, deplete bile flow, damage the gut lining, and trigger long-term digestive dysfunction. I didn't learn that until years later, when I was already dealing with chronic inflammation, bile sluggishness, and liver markers that kept raising red flags.

I wasn't warned. I wasn't told what to look for. I was just handed a prescription and told it would clear my skin. It did clear my skin. But it also set off a chain reaction that took years to manifest.

Looking back, Accutane was my first lesson in the hidden costs of modern medicine. Not the acute side effects listed in fine print, but the slow, silent disruption of systems that are foundational to health: detoxification, digestion, hormonal balance. I had no idea how vital those systems were until mine were no longer working right.

And I feared I was on the same path as all the Wilson men before me. Each one gone too soon. Worse, I felt betrayed by the experts. Was this it? A lifetime of symptom management and no real answers? I started to wonder if "healthcare" had anything to do with health at all.

Then came a dinner that changed everything. I was sitting with my father-in-law and his friend JT. The topic turned to my degree in health sciences and the mess my own health had become. JT listened, paused, then said, "You need to see my doctor."

He wasn't talking about another specialist. He described a doctor who taught people how to heal. He explained how the nervous system governs every function of the body, yet nearly every "healthcare" solution disrupts and interferes with the system. He didn't believe in suppressing symptoms. He taught his patients to uncover root causes.

I had never heard health described this way. And I had never seen someone speak about a doctor with such conviction. I reached out. He became a mentor. A guide. And for the first time, I saw a new path forward. One that didn't just manage disease but restored function.

That year, my symptoms disappeared. But something deeper happened. I experienced what it meant to heal. And I saw that healing isn't a destination. It's a state of being.

That shift changed everything. I realized my healing wasn't just for me. I was being called to help others reclaim theirs. Over the next four years, I devoured everything I could get my hands on related to nervous system optimization. Chiropractic adjustments, nutrition, detoxification, movement, mindset. I was obsessed. I didn't just want to "have a career" in natural health, I wanted to change the way people viewed and managed their health and healthcare. I wanted them to experience a life free from fear and the bondage that comes with traditional methods.

But head knowledge wasn't enough. As a former athlete, I knew the difference between knowing and owning something. I needed training. So I moved to Naples, Florida, to train under one of the brightest minds in natural health and chiropractic, Dr. Joel Bohemier.

Eight years of postgrad education were already behind me. I didn't move because I needed another credential. I moved to fulfill a God-given dream to help people exit medicine and build a life that produces vitality. I didn't know it at the time, but Naples became the fertile ground that allowed the vision to blossom.

Now and for over a decade in private practice, I've helped tens of thousands of people break free from the cycle of symptom management and reclaim their vitality. Our clinic became one of the largest natural health centers in the country. Not because of ads or marketing budgets, but because people got real results and shared it.

I've traveled the country teaching the principles of health and healing. I speak to moms, dads, doctors, and health leaders. The multiplication effect is real. And this book is part of that multiplication. It's meant to give you the same tools, frameworks, and truth I wish someone had handed me when I was eighteen and falling apart.

I use the word "vitality" a lot, and you'll soon see why. But here's what you need to know right now. Whether you're battling a chronic diagnosis or just want to raise healthy kids in a toxic world, the human body was designed to heal. When every system is firing, every cell repairing, and every choice is aligned with the design, that's vitality. And you were made for it.

Our family is united by a shared mission: helping individuals reclaim their health freedom and, in doing so, empowering entire families to do the same. This mission would not exist without my wife, Leah. She's not just my partner in life; she's a force in both policy and advocacy, reshaping how health is viewed and managed from grassroots gatherings of mothers and fathers to national debates about medical freedom.

With that, I will hand the page to Leah. We are writing this book together, and our mission wouldn't exist without her story and experience.

Leah: When Fighting for Families Means Fighting the System

From a young age, I saw firsthand how broken systems harm the very people they claim to help. It shaped everything about the way I see justice, freedom, and what it truly means to advocate for those without a voice.

I never set out to work in health freedom. My original passion was child advocacy. I wanted to fix the foster care system, to create a world where kids didn't age out without a family to call their own, where vulnerable children weren't medicated into submission because the system lacked the will to provide real care. I saw too many kids diagnosed with "disorders" that were really just symptoms of trauma, neglect, and a desperate need for love.

I pursued law hoping that I could help change the system from within. I had every intention of working in child welfare, fighting for better outcomes for foster kids. But when I applied for a job at the Indiana Department of Child Services, despite graduating near the top of my class, I was denied the opportunity. It was my first taste of just how uninterested the system was in being fixed.

So I took a different path. I found myself in big law, working on high-stakes corporate litigation, bet-the-company cases that would make or break massive industries. And I loved it. I thrived in it. The partners I worked with were among the best legal minds in the country, and I was on the path to an incredible career.

But then, our own family was caught in the very kind of government overreach I had spent years fighting against. Nick and I were already foster-ing children, opening our home to kids in need. It wasn't just something we did, it was part of who we were. We had been through the process before, and we were preparing to renew our foster license when I received an email that stopped me in my tracks: The state of Indiana requires proof that your biological children are up to date on their required vaccinations. I simply resubmitted our religious exemption, just as we had done in pre-vious years. But this time was different. The agency responded: The state will not accept your exemption. Unvaccinated children in the household are a "threat to the welfare" of foster children.

I read the words over and over again. Our healthy children were now a threat? It didn't make sense. It wasn't logical. And it certainly wasn't sci-ence. I pushed back, escalating the issue through every channel available. I demanded an explanation, citing the law, the evidence, and the absurdity of their stance.

But the response was firm: *Either comply, or your foster license will be permanently revoked.* I was furious. Not just for us, but for the children who would now be denied a safe home because of a shortage of foster homes combined with a nonsensical policy. Nick and I looked at each other and asked, *Where do we go from here?*

We had signed up to help foster children in a time of need. Now, we were watching those same children suffer at the hands of bad policies driven by politics, not common sense. We made a decision that night. If we weren't allowed to help these kids quietly, we would educate and empower enough people that this kind of injustice couldn't continue. That's how our nonprofit, Stand for Health Freedom, was born.

Six years later, we've mobilized almost one million people, helped defeat harmful laws, advanced pro-health reforms, and stopped govern-ment overreach in its tracks. Parents, doctors, and everyday citizens are standing together to fight for the right to make health decisions without fear, pressure, or government interference.

Nick again: Leah's story is just as much a part of this book as mine. We've spent years on the front lines of health and freedom, and now we're bringing everything we've learned to you. Together, we want to empower you with the tools, the knowledge, and the conviction to reclaim your health, your family's health, and your freedom. We wrote this book together, but you'll often come across the word "I" as we've decided on narrating through my voice.

But our fight for health freedom isn't just about personal battles; it's about a larger crisis unfolding all around us. The more we pushed back against the system, the more we realized these weren't just policy failures or bureaucratic overreach. They were symptoms of a much deeper issue: an entire culture of health that has been turned upside down.

Chronic disease has been normalized. Dependence on pharmaceuticals has been celebrated. Natural health practices, the very things that sustained human beings for generations, have been dismissed as fringe or even dangerous. Meanwhile, the bodies of men, women, and children are breaking down at an unprecedented rate.

This isn't just about flawed policies or corrupt institutions. It's about the survival of a species.

The Bigger Picture: A Species in Decline

The failures we fought against weren't isolated incidents, they were symptoms of a much bigger crisis. We are facing an existential threat to human health:

- Chronic disease now kills 8 out of 10 people in industrialized nations (Eaton et al., "Stone Agers in the Fast Lane").
- US birth rates have dropped from 123 per 1,000 women in 1957 to 55 in 2023 (USA Facts).
- More than half of Americans have at least one chronic disease.
- Neurological disorders are surging—autism rates have skyrocketed from 1 in 150 in 2000 to 1 in 31 today.

The decline isn't just medical, it's societal. Seventy percent of military-aged men are unfit to serve. We are quite literally becoming too sick to defend ourselves. And yet, instead of asking why this is happening, Medicine's only answer is more drugs (even personalized drugs), more procedures, and more dependence. Morally we cannot continue on this same path. Financially our country is in trouble, with the rise in healthcare costs outpacing the rise in GDP. There is a way out. You are a part of it. It will require a paradigm shift, something more than just swapping chemical treatments for natural treatments and something more than simply using preventative testing.

But the good news is this: health freedom is still in your hands.

Once you understand how the body is designed to heal and adapt, you'll have a blueprint for making clear, confident health decisions, ones that remove you from the cycle of chronic illness and dependence. The only real solution to reversing the chronic disease pandemic isn't another medication, another specialist, or another government policy. It's a fundamental shift in how we view and pursue health.

Where We Go from Here?

- In part 1, we'll expose the broken healthcare system and why it's time to exit conventional Medicine.
- In part 2, we'll reveal the real causes of chronic illness including nervous system dysregulation, toxicity, and environmental stressors.
- In part 3, we'll explore how to reclaim your health by aligning with natural laws of healing, balancing your nervous system, and regaining health freedom.

The journey back to health isn't about finding the next trend or hack, it's about trusting the blueprint your body already has.

Disclaimer: The authors are not involved in Medicine, they do not practice Medicine, nor do they desire any association with Medicine. This book is intended to serve as an informational guide, and its core purpose is to help you make truly informed decisions about your health.

PART I

Exit Conventional Medicine

To reclaim vitality, you have to first understand what it is: Vitality is the fullness of life; the inborn capacity to heal. There are three principles of vitality. The first is simple: **Your body was designed to heal.**

Healing isn't the exception. It's the default "programming" of every function of the human body. It's the *natural* state. And I emphasize "natural" for a reason. You've been told that natural is an alternative to medical intervention. That there's only one path to health, the conventional medical model. That model doesn't just ignore "natural." It rejects it, mocks it, and attempts to relegate it to the fringes of society and classify it as reckless. All you have to do to test this theory is simply mention "natural cures" to your doctor and watch their body language shift. It's not just skepticism. It's disdain.

The first principle of vitality is to remind you that quite the opposite is true about health: medical intervention is an alternative to supporting the intricacy and brilliance of the God-given design of the human body.

If we want to reclaim our birthright, vitality, we have to stop outsourcing our "healthcare" to a system that rejects the foundations of health and healing.

That requires a paradigm shift in the way that we think about health, symptoms, and health decisions. It is a necessary shift if we want to reverse the horrible trends of unnecessary human suffering. That's what part 1 is all about: the case for exiting the playing field of conventional Medicine.

CHAPTER 1

The Body Is Brilliant

Humans are an animal species. We have a genetically determined required habitat and lifestyle, just like every other species. If we live outside of this required habitat and lifestyle, we get sick—just like every other species does when taken out of its natural environment.

—Dr. James Chestnut

The Backpack Analogy by Dr. James Chestnut: Why We're Sinking

Imagine you're born floating in water with a backpack and a built-in flotation device that has a pinhole. The slow, steady loss of air through that hole represents natural aging. In an ideal state, your backpack stays light enough to keep you afloat, moving through life with energy, clarity, and resilience. But as life happens, rocks, such as stress, toxins, injuries, and other burdens, begin to fill your backpack.

Every rock added along the way makes the backpack heavier, and as the weight increases, staying afloat becomes harder. Most people aren't drowning because they're deficient in pharmaceutical drugs; they're drowning because their backpack is too heavy.

Fight or Flight versus Rest and Repair

The nervous system is your body's adaptive intelligence. It is the system responsible for adjusting to the inevitable weight of your backpack. But every rock you add affects its ability to adapt. Even a healthy nervous system has a limit. When it is functioning well, it can recalibrate, recover, and keep you afloat. But the more it is burdened, the harder it is to bounce back. It is the control center for healing, regulation, and response. And when it is dysregulated, no amount of diet, exercise, or supplements will bring back vitality. That is the piece missing from most health strategies, including functional medicine.

Your nervous system has two primary states:

- **Sympathetic (fight or flight)**: The stress response, designed for short-term survival.
- **Parasympathetic (rest and repair)**: The healing state, where digestion, regeneration, and immune function thrive.

In the wild, animals experience stress in short bursts. A gazelle runs from a lion. A bird dodges a predator. Then, the nervous system shifts back into recovery mode. Humans, on the other hand, are stuck in perpetual overdrive. Constant deadlines, endless notifications, poor sleep, financial strain, processed foods, and fear-driven health narratives, this is captivity. And when the nervous system is stuck in stress mode, healing is put on hold.

Most conventional treatments add more rocks to the backpack. Another prescription, another suppressive therapy, when in reality, what the body actually needs is to remove interference and restore nervous system balance.

A Captive Species

Years ago, I was standing in front of the tiger exhibit at the zoo with my two sons. The younger one was pressed up against the glass, eyes wide with wonder, captivated by the size and strength of the tigers just a few feet away from him. The tigers paced back and forth, muscles rippling beneath their striped coats. On the surface, they looked powerful. But the zookeeper's words painted a different picture.

"These tigers are healthy enough to survive," she explained, "but captivity takes a toll. Their fertility rates are lower, they're more prone to illness, and their behavior doesn't match what you'd see in the wild."

She went on to describe the specifics: captivity stifled their instincts, their nutrition was artificial, and chronic stress weakened their immune systems. "They're missing what makes them wild," she said. Her words stuck with me. The tigers were alive, but they weren't thriving.

We often marvel at wild animals, recognizing that when a creature is removed from its natural environment, its health and behavior decline. We don't question this when it comes to animals. But when it comes to humans, we've convinced ourselves that we're the exception.

We wake up to alarms instead of sunrise. We stare at screens instead of firelight. We sit in traffic instead of walking under open skies. We are overstimulated, undernourished, and overburdened. And then we wonder why our bodies feel broken.

Our ancestors moved in natural environments, nourished their bodies with whole foods, lived deeply connected to family and faith, and experienced stress in short bursts that strengthened them. Our bodies thrived in that environment because we were designed for it. We don't live wild anymore. We live in captivity. And just like animals in captivity, our bodies are breaking down as a result.

The Body as a Masterpiece

The good news is that, despite everything we've done to deviate from our natural design, the human body remains a resilient masterpiece. Your body is not a machine that needs constant tinkering; it is a highly intelligent, self-regulating, self-healing system. Your body is fighting for you, not against you. Take a moment to think about the next paragraphs.

Every second of every day, your body is working tirelessly on your behalf, fighting to regenerate and heal. Without you even noticing, it's orchestrating millions of intricate processes, each one vital to your survival. Your heart beats over 100,000 times a day, pumping blood to deliver oxygen and nutrients to every cell. Your lungs expand and contract thousands of times to draw in life-giving air. Even when you're asleep, your body is repairing tissues, processing memories, and regulating hormones. It never stops; it was created to serve you.

Your skin is a marvel. It is your first line of defense against the outside world, constantly renewing to stay strong and resilient. About every month, most of the cells in its outermost layer are replaced, forming a fresh barrier to protect you from harm. Beneath that surface, your bones are just as remarkable. After a break, they repair and remodel along lines of stress, often returning stronger where the load is greatest. This precision design is written into your biology, maximizing your chances of survival.

Consider your liver, often taken for granted yet capable of astonishing feats. Even after losing up to 75 percent of its mass, your liver can regenerate itself, restoring its ability to detoxify your blood, produce essential proteins, and store vital nutrients. These are purposeful, deliberate processes designed to keep you alive and thriving.

The human brain processes millions of pieces of information every second, regulates bodily functions, stores memories, and enables complex thought, creativity, and emotions. The phenomenon of consciousness, our ability to be self-aware and think abstractly, is one of the greatest mysteries and marvels of the body.

The same intelligence that heals a broken bone also regulates your hormones, digests your food, and keeps you alive.

The Greatest Doctor Is Already Inside You

When you scrape your knee, you don't have to tell your body how to clot blood, repair skin, or fight off infection. It just happens. When you have a cold, your body raises its temperature, increases immune cell production, and mounts an attack against any potential invaders. Your body is continually orchestrating millions of intricate processes, all with one goal: survival and adaptation.

Take a fever, for example. We're conditioned to see it as a problem, something to be suppressed. But a fever isn't a failure. It's your body's way of burning off infection. Or consider inflammation: it's not the enemy; it's a coordinated response, your body sending reinforcements to heal an injury. Yet, instead of supporting these processes, we suppress them. We take drugs to bring down fevers, medications to mute inflammation, and chemicals to numb pain, all without ever asking why these symptoms are happening in the first place. What is your body trying to tell you?

Instead of constantly trying to manipulate the body, more often we simply need to get out of the way. Your body isn't a problem to be solved;

it's a masterpiece to be supported. Your job is to trust it and give it the conditions it needs to thrive. When we stop trying to outsmart the body, we begin to unlock its full potential.

Freedom from Interference

Healing isn't forced; it happens when you stop getting in the way. Your body is wired to heal, but it cannot do its job amid constant interference. We interfere at every turn: chronic stress, processed food, chemical exposure, fear. Like the tigers kept outside their natural habitat, we do not thrive in the wrong conditions.

Your body hasn't failed you. The problem is the interference that disrupts its design. Live in alignment with your God-given design, and healing follows.

And that brings us to a crucial concept: healing is not about adding more. Healing happens when we remove what is blocking the body from doing what it was created to do. Your body doesn't need more, it needs less interference.

What is your body trying to tell you? Instead of trying to outsmart the body, we need to start listening. Your body isn't a problem to be solved, it's a masterpiece to be supported. Your job is to trust the design and give it the conditions it needs to thrive.

We live in a culture obsessed with fixing and optimizing, but the more we tinker with the body's design, the more unintended consequences we create. Man's knowledge is limited, and even well-intended interventions can disrupt the intricate systems we barely understand.

Most health books tell you what to eat, what supplement to take, or what habits to build. All of those things matter, but they won't get you the breakthrough or results you are looking for without the inclusion of this foundational principle of health:

Your nervous system decides whether your body adapts to stress or breaks down under it.

Trust the Design

Vitality isn't something you have to chase; it's something you were created to experience. This is the foundation of vitality. And this is where your journey back to true health begins.

There are some who have tried every diet, every protocol, and every supplement, yet are still exhausted, inflamed, and stuck. That's often because they haven't addressed the root cause: a dysregulated nervous system.

This book will show you how to remove interference, regulate your nervous system, and return to the state of vitality that is your birthright. This doesn't mean abandoning modern life. It means rewilding your health by embracing principles that support vitality.

The Path Forward

You are not broken. Your body is not against you. And you don't need another complicated health strategy to unlock vitality. You need to rethink everything you've been told.

- What if you trusted your body more than you trusted the experts?
- What if health isn't something you chase but something you allow?
- What if the only thing standing between you and vitality . . . is interference?

This is the path to reclaim your vitality. In the next chapter, we address how we have been taught that the prudent thing to do in time of physical need is to consult with your doctor. It is imperative that you consult with experts and authorities that you trust. Otherwise, the framework that even world-class experts work within can become more of a cost than a benefit.

CHAPTER 2

Conventional Medicine: More than Broken

It is simply no longer possible to believe much of the clinical research that is published, or to rely on the judgment of trusted physicians or authoritative medical guidelines. I take no pleasure in this conclusion, which I reached slowly and reluctantly over my two decades as an editor.
—Dr. Marcia Angell (former editor in chief of
The New England Journal of Medicine)

Mr. Pryor showed up with joint pain, brain fog, fatigue, and dizziness so intense he had to grip the counter when standing to talk to my team at the front desk. Fifteen prescriptions lined his daily pillbox, each one meant to manage the side effects of the last. He thought he was treating different conditions. But what he was really experiencing was a chain reaction created by the system itself.

His blood pressure meds caused dizziness. The statins worsened his joint pain. His pain relievers spiked his blood pressure again. When we reviewed his full list, it was clear. He was being drugged to death.

This is not an unusual story. It's become the norm. It's what I call the medical merry-go-round. A place where the solution to every new symptom is another pill, and the underlying problems are never addressed. The ride doesn't end with healing. It ends with dependency, deterioration, and often, death.

So the question is worth asking: why is this accepted as normal?

In this book, you'll notice that I capitalize Medicine. That's intentional. Medicine, as I refer to it here, is not the practice of getting sick people well; it is the medical-industrial complex, a system driven by profit, bureaucracy, and control, rather than true healing. There is a stark difference between the art of medicine, practiced by those genuinely seeking to restore health, and Medicine, the monopolized industry that dictates protocols (i.e., "standard of care") and pushes pharmaceuticals and the barbaric practice of removing organs, resulting in more pharmaceuticals to support artificial functions and keeps people trapped in chronic illness.

Medicine: The Leading Cause of Death

We are told that heart disease and cancer are America's top killers, with medical error a distant third.[1] That is the official story. Pause and ask how those numbers are assembled. What gets left out is more alarming than what makes the list.

When mainstream sources say "medicine is the third leading cause of death," they are talking mainly about iatrogenesis (harm caused by medical care), such as surgical mistakes, wrong prescriptions, and bad drug reactions.[2] Those numbers are shocking, but they leave out a larger issue: the overall harm caused by Medicine as an industry.

If we widen the lens beyond just medical error, we see a much more damning picture. When researchers calculate the total burden of medical harm, they include:

1. **Nosocomial infections (hospital-acquired infections)** kill over 100,000 people annually. Yet, they are excluded from iatrogenic death statistics, despite being a direct consequence of hospitalization.

2. **Polypharmacy-induced (caused by taking multiple medications at the same time) death and chronic deterioration:** Millions of people take medications not to heal but to manage the side effects of other medications, leading to slow, uncounted deaths from organ failure, suppressed immunity, and metabolic collapse.

3. **Iatrogenic harm (harm caused by medical care) beyond medical error:** Deaths caused not by an underlying illness, but by the prescribed treatment itself, such as chemotherapy toxicity, unnecessary surgeries, and adverse pharmaceutical interactions.[3, 4, 5]

The more powerful the drugs become, the more dangerous they are.

Let me give you some examples: a person is told they need a statin to control their cholesterol so they don't have a heart attack. What they aren't told is that statins wreak havoc on muscle and neurological function, leaving patients frail, immobile, and vulnerable. A person is told they need psychiatric medications to have a meaningful life because of prolonged and deep sadness. What they are not told is that this class of drugs creates a dependency cycle that alters brain chemistry permanently and cuts off connection to the outside world and other people that you love by dampening your emotions.[6]

And then, there's the mass-casualty event that no one in Medicine wants to account for: the COVID era.

Never before had an experimental technology been rushed to market at "warp speed"and mandated on an unsuspecting public without long-term safety data. The mRNA injections were not just a medical intervention; they were a social experiment on a scale never seen before. Adverse events were dismissed and overtly censored by government influence and tech cooperation,[7, 8] concerns were deleted from history, and the bodies piled up, yet somehow these deaths don't make it into the statistics on medical harm. Why? Because when a treatment is widely accepted as "safe and effective," any damage it causes gets rebranded as coincidence even by the overseeing experts themselves.

Dr. Lucian Leape, a Harvard professor, exposed that Medicine kills the equivalent of three jumbo jets' worth of American patients every forty-eight hours.[9] She made this statement in 1994; it's exponentially worse now.[10] This is not a minor flaw in the system; it is a crisis, even fraud.

Medicine's Saving Grace: Crisis and Emergency Care

If there's one place where modern Medicine shines, it's in crisis care. When you're in the middle of a heart attack, when your appendix ruptures, when you're pulled from a car wreck with multiple fractures, there is no replacement for the tools of emergency Medicine. The ability to stabilize a trauma patient, perform lifesaving surgeries, and manage acute infections with precision is a true medical achievement. In life-or-death situations, the medical model can do extraordinary things. This is where Medicine thrives.

The problem isn't what Medicine can do in a crisis; it's what happens when that crisis model governs everyday health care. It also happens when the body's warning signs and symptoms are sold as a "crisis" or an "emergency." Every chronic condition, from diabetes to high blood pressure to autoimmune disease, is managed as if it were an emergency. Drugs are prescribed to suppress symptoms, or procedures are performed to remove the affected tissue.

But within Medicine, no thought is given to the root causes, and there is no respect for the body's intelligent communication to you through the expression of symptoms. Even worse, there is no consideration for the long-term impact. Medicine applies the same high-intervention, high-cost methods to everyday health problems, turning routine care into an ongoing cycle of medical dependency. It has evolved into a radical monopoly, not just controlling treatment, but dictating public policy, medical education, and even what a doctor is allowed to communicate or offer to his patients.

Medicine and healthcare at large are sadly no longer about healing; it is a principal economic activity, legitimizing a system that keeps people sick and dependent. This shift didn't happen by accident. To understand how Medicine became an industry built on profit rather than restoration, we need to look at its origins.

How Did We Get Here?

To understand how Medicine became a monopoly, we must look at one of its most powerful architects of the system: the Rockefeller Foundation. Established in 1913, this institution has played an outsized role in shaping the modern medical landscape.[11] Its influence on healthcare has been both far-reaching and devastating.

One of its most significant impacts was the promotion of Medicine (the allopathic model of diagnosing, treating and preventing illnesses) at the expense of traditional and natural healing methods.[12] By funding research and medical schools that focused solely on pharmaceuticals and surgery, the Rockefeller Foundation ensured that alternative approaches, such as chiropractic, naturopathy, and nutritional healing, were sidelined, dismissed, or outright eliminated.[13] This is no conjecture or hearsay or observation. It is all readily discoverable in the plan laid out in the Flexner Report.[14]

The Flexner Report and the Eradication of Medical Diversity

A defining moment in the monopolization of Medicine was the Flexner Report of 1910, which the Rockefeller Foundation helped push forward.[15] This report evaluated medical schools across the United States and Canada, but rather than improving all forms of healthcare, it set a new standard that heavily favored allopathic Medicine. The result is that countless medical schools teaching homeopathy, herbal Medicine, and holistic care were shut down.[16] Meanwhile, schools that embraced drug-based, high-intervention Medicine were elevated.[17]

The impact of this was profound:

- Medical education became standardized around pharmaceuticals and surgery.
- Natural healing practices were systematically erased from mainstream Medicine.
- The pharmaceutical industry gained a stranglehold on healthcare, as the new medical system depended almost entirely on patented drugs.[18]

Medicine for Profit, Not for Healing

The Rockefeller Foundation's heavy investment in the pharmaceutical industry was no coincidence. The family name was well-known for the success of Standard Oil. Rockefeller saw an opportunity to monetize healthcare by promoting pharmaceutical medicine because it could be built on petroleum-based products. His empire had already conquered the energy industry. So turning crude oil by-products into medical treatments would allow him to take on a new sector: pharmaceuticals.[19] The concept of treating every illness with a corresponding pill became the dominant model largely due to the influence of John D. Rockefeller.

Consider the overuse of antibiotics: While these drugs can be lifesaving in acute cases, the Rockefeller-backed model encouraged their widespread and indiscriminate use. The result? An epidemic of antibiotic-resistant bacteria that has created new, man-made plagues.[20] This is a problem recognized by Medicine.[21] Moreover, the health crisis is fueled by the atomic bomb that antibiotics and other chemical interferences have been on the microbiome, leading to untold cancers and metabolic dysfunction.[22]

The uptake in use of drugs was not a coincidence. It was an intentional design fueled by economic strategy.

The Illusion of Progress

For over a century, Western Medicine has written the story that its advancements have single-handedly extended human life.[23] The medical-industrial complex paints itself as the architect of longer, healthier lives, but the data tells a different story. The sharp decline in mortality from infectious diseases like scarlet fever, diphtheria, and measles occurred before the introduction of antibiotics and vaccines.[24] The historical data shows that the real heroes of increased longevity are improved sanitation, better nutrition, and cleaner living environments, none of which were Medical innovations.[25] The pharmaceutical industry didn't save us; nature and improved living conditions did.[26]

Despite this, the allopathic model took credit for progress it did not create. It doubled down on its claim as the sole authority on health while failing to address the rise of modern chronic diseases. Heart disease, diabetes, obesity, autoimmune conditions, and mental disorders now plague society at unprecedented levels.[27] These are not infectious illnesses solved with a pill or a vaccine; they are the consequences of a society that has been misled into believing that health comes in a prescription bottle. The more Medicine "advanced," the sicker people became.

Medicine has had its heyday now for over a century and has spent trillions of dollars to prove its effectiveness, yet survival rates for the most common cancers have barely budged in decades.[28] The five-year survival rate for breast cancer is still only 50 percent, regardless of screening frequency or treatment methods.[29] Billions have been spent since President Richard Nixon declared the war on cancer in 1971.[30] The most heavily funded medical research has failed to produce meaningful improvements, yet the industry continues to claim itself as the only legitimate option. The truth is, the allopathic model was never designed to cure or restore health. It was built to measure, diagnose, and manage disease. Most people stay trapped in its cycle of interventions. Not because they are getting well, but because they are told they have no other choice. "It's genetic." "It's better than doing nothing." "You have to."

Medicine Is Incompatible with Health Restoration

This is where the system reveals its fundamental flaw. It is not designed or purposed to rebuild health. It does not ask why a person became sick in the first place. It only seeks to manage, suppress, and intervene, and all of its tools follow that aim.

And yet, Medicine has positioned itself not just as one tool among many, but as the only legitimate authority on health. It has become, in many ways, a belief system. A structure of control. A monolithic institution that tolerates no alternatives. But once you see how Medicine has taken on the role of the one true faith of health, it changes everything. This is medical monotheism.

Medical Monotheism: The One True Faith of Modern Medicine

Over time, Medicine has positioned itself not merely as science, but as a belief system that tolerates no competing perspectives. It has become medical monotheism: the doctrine that there is only one true path to health, and that path runs exclusively through the institutions of Medicine.

Like any monotheistic faith, medical monotheism has its central authorities: the high priests of health in the form of the CDC, FDA, WHO, and pharmaceutical industry. It has its sacred texts: guidelines and studies that are treated as unquestionable, even when they are riddled with corporate influence. It has its missionaries: doctors, nurses, educators and scientists who are trained to spread its gospel. And it has its heretics: those who dare to challenge its teachings and, in doing so, face professional and social excommunication.[31]

We've been raised in this system. So we often fail to recognize it for what it is. From the moment we are born, we are conditioned to *believe in* Medicine. The white coat is a symbol of authority. The prescription pad is a sacred scroll. The vaccine schedule is an unchallenged rite of passage. Even the language is religious. Doctors deliver us from disease. Medicine saves lives. Anyone who dares to question it is labeled "anti-science."[32]

Many Christians, even those who deeply trust in God, still believe that Medicine is a "gift from God." And in many ways, that's true. Medical advancements have undeniably saved lives. But what if that gift has been hijacked? What if what was once a tool for healing has become a system of control? What if that tool of control has numbed and extinguished our respect for God's brilliant design of our bodies? Treating the human body as if it is defective and broken and putting more faith in a spoonful of medicine than the power that animates the living world doesn't add up when you look at Medicine's track record. Our children deserve better.

If you don't hold to a biblical worldview, you can still reclaim vitality. Truth is truth, regardless of belief. But in my experience, those with faith are often more resistant to the lies and manipulation of Medicine because they recognize that health isn't man-made; it's God-given. And yet, even among believers, there are beliefs that keep them tethered to the medical system. Many place more faith in pharmaceuticals than in the body's design, accepting medical intervention as inevitable rather than considering whether it aligns with the design.

Pharmakia: The Gift from God?

The Greek word *pharmakia*, from which we get "pharmaceutical," appears multiple times in Scripture. It is never used in a positive light.

In Galatians 5:19–21, pharmakia is listed among the "works of the flesh" that lead to destruction, translated as sorcery or witchcraft.[33] Revelation 18:23 warns that "the nations were deceived by your sorcery (pharmakia)": a prophecy that seems eerily relevant in an age where billions are conditioned to believe that health and miracles can only come from pharmaceutical intervention.[34]

The Bible's warnings about pharmakia were not just about potions and spells: they were about manipulation, deception, and control through mind-altering substances. What is modern Medicine if not the globalized, industrialized fulfillment of this very concept?

Look at the opioid crisis. Pharmaceutical companies knowingly pushed addictive painkillers on the population, destroying millions of lives, all while assuring the public that these drugs were safe.[35] Look at the psychiatric industry, where millions are placed on antidepressants, antipsychotics, and mood stabilizers, trapped in cycles of dependence while their conditions worsen over time.[36] Look at the COVID era, where an experimental injection was forced upon entire populations under the guise of salvation, and those who resisted were demonized.[37]

This is the reality of modern *pharmakia*. It promises healing but delivers harm. It claims to save but enslaves instead. But if this is really about science, then where is the debate? Science, by definition, requires constant questioning, challenging, and refining of ideas. But in medical monotheism, questioning is not allowed. Dissent is not tolerated. Alternative perspectives are ridiculed, silenced, and, in some cases, outright banned.

And yet, many people of faith still defend the system, arguing that we *need* Medicine because we live in a "fallen world," as if our bodies were designed to be sick from birth, forever dependent on pharmaceuticals to function properly. But recognizing that we live in a fallen world simply means acknowledging that our bodies will break down over time, not that sickness is our default state or that we are powerless to resist it. The Bible doesn't teach that disease is inevitable and unmanageable. Rather, it teaches stewardship. We are called to honor and care for our bodies, not surrender them to a system dependent on their decline.

The "fallen world" argument is too often used as a passive justification for sickness. It's used as a scapegoat to justify the existence of a disease while accepting the next pharmaceutical intervention without question. But this thinking is built on a flawed belief: that the body is destined for dysfunction, and drugs are the only way to survive. This ignores the fact that our bodies were fearfully and wonderfully made, designed with resilience, adaptability, and the ability to heal. It removes the questions and curiosity of what might have caused the sickness in the first place. It also strips away faith in God's provision, replacing it with faith in a system that thrives on keeping people dependent.

Yes, we live in a world where things go wrong, but that doesn't mean we were created to be sick or that we should default to pharmaceutical solutions as our only hope. Medicine is not a savior. The body is not the enemy. And faith doesn't mean abandoning the responsibility to steward our health. It means trusting that true healing comes through alignment with God's design, not through a lifetime of artificial intervention.

The Dogma of the "One True Path"

There is a reason medical monotheism thrives: it keeps people dependent. When Medicine is treated as the only path to health, nutrition, lifestyle, and toxicity are pushed aside as irrelevant or dismissed as unscientific. If disease is something that happens to you, something you "catch" or "get," then you are a passive victim in need of medical intervention, not an active participant in your health. If the only solution to illness comes from a prescription or a procedure, then you will always need Medicine, and Medicine will always have control.

This model does not promote health. It promotes compliance. And when people do get sick, rather than questioning the system itself, they blame themselves for not following the medical commandments well enough. "I should have taken my statin." "I should have gotten my flu shot." "I should have gone to the doctor sooner." The system never considers that maybe the very interventions it prescribes are part of the problem.

Faith-Based, Not Evidence-Based

Medicine is presented as objective, rational, and above reproach. But belief in Medicine often operates in the absence of true evidence, or even in direct contradiction to it.

Take the rapid adoption of cholesterol-lowering drugs. For decades, statins have been prescribed to lower cholesterol and prevent heart disease. The problem? The entire premise, that cholesterol causes heart disease, has been challenged by extensive research, yet the guidelines remain unchanged.[38] Why? Because Medicine is not about evidence; it's about maintaining control.

Or look at antibiotics. We were told they were one of the greatest medical breakthroughs, yet decades of overprescription have led to antibiotic resistance, destroying gut microbiomes and creating new diseases in the process.[39] Still, antibiotics remain a go-to solution for even minor infections, and sometimes those that are viral like the routine antibiotic prescription for childhood ear infections. This is notable because of the overuse, but also because antibiotics are used to treat bacterial infections like strep throat or urinary tract infections. They are not effective against viral illnesses.

And then there's the most glaring example of all: the COVID-19 response. The public was promised that the mRNA injections were "safe and effective," despite the lack of long-term data, despite the rushed development, and despite the mounting reports of injury. Any hesitation was condemned. Any dissenting voices were silenced. The entire world was subjected to a mass experiment under the guise of scientific certainty. And yet, Medicine refuses to look back and acknowledge its mistakes.

If Medicine were truly about evidence, we would see adjustments, apologies, and massive reform. But the reform is not coming any time soon. Even as the market demands have increased in the post-COVID era.

The Pandemic Awakening

The good news is that people are waking up. A record number of individuals are seeking alternative health solutions, questioning the necessity of lifelong medication, and recognizing the glaring holes in the allopathic model. Functional Medicine, chiropractic care, and holistic approaches are surging in popularity, not because of clever marketing, government recommendations or school mandates, but because they work.

If there was ever a moment that pulled back the curtain, it was the pandemic. People who had never questioned the medical system before suddenly saw it for what it was. They witnessed the rigid enforcement of "one-size-fits-all" Medicine, the suppression of alternative viewpoints, and the blatant prioritization of industry interests over individual health.[40]

For the first time, many people asked:

- Can you help me find a natural pediatrician?
- Do you know a good holistic MD who won't force the shot?

They began searching for alternatives, realizing that the allopathic system had failed them. But as time has gone on, more people are realizing that they don't just want a doctor who will give a more natural form of medication—they desire doctors who are "awake." They want a doctor who will empower them to make their own healthcare decisions. They desire an approach that produces energy and vitality, not addictions and dependence. Yet, asking this from Medicine has proved to be a tall task.

For the first time there is evidence that the American public is ready to break free from medical monotheism. Recognizing this truth is not about rejecting Medicine altogether. It is about putting Medicine back in its place. Medicine should be a tool, one of many, not the only one. It should be subject to scrutiny, not above it. It should serve humanity, not rule over it.

If we want to reclaim our health, we must break free from this system of blind faith. We must stop outsourcing our bodies to an institution that sees us as patients, as broken and defective, not as people in a symbiotic relationship with our environment and brilliantly designed to heal.

Because health does not come from a prescription pad. It comes from within.

The Cure Is a Mirage

"Searching for the cure" to chronic, lifestyle-induced diseases is one of the most profitable distractions ever manufactured. Doctors chase it, scientists chase it, and the public clings to it like salvation, believing that one day a miracle drug will save them from the consequences of how they live. But it won't. Because the system doesn't want it to.[41]

The majority of today's chronic illnesses, including heart disease, type 2 diabetes, neurodegenerative conditions like Alzheimer's, autoimmune disorders, and nearly all forms of cancer, aren't random acts of fate or result of a "fallen world." They are the predictable outcome of how we eat, move, think, sleep, and live. These diseases are constructed, not caught. And yet, the pharmaceutical industry keeps you focused on the wrong target. It prioritizes treatment over cause and symptom suppression over restoration.

Even if a pharmaceutical "cure" were possible—and from a vitalistic perspective it is not—the concept of a cure threatens the entire medical business model. Healing removes the need for the system. Reversal ends the revenue stream. That is why the model is not built around cures. It is built around customers.

Take the example that is often cited as a breakthrough "cure." In 2015, Gilead Sciences released a new drug for hepatitis C. It worked by their standards of measurement, it knocked down the viral response. Patients tested negative for the virus after treatment. By conventional metrics, it was called a cure.[42] Even though halting or silencing a virus is not the same as restoring health, and from a vitalistic lens, this was not a true cure because it only muted the symptom (more on this in the next chapter), Gilead's drug appeared to work. And because people were no longer "sick," they no longer needed the drug. Within two years, Gilead's revenue dropped by more than ten billion dollars.[43]

Goldman Sachs took notice. In a 2018 biotech research report, they asked a blunt question: Is curing patients a sustainable business model? Their answer was clear. One-shot cures may sound attractive in theory, but they undermine recurring revenue.[44] In plain language, healing people is bad for business.

That's not a conspiracy theory. That's a financial analysis. When the system is built on recurring sickness, cures become a threat. Real healing undermines the entire business model. And so the focus remains on life-long dependency on drugs, specialists, and systems that promise management but never restoration.

If we know how these diseases are built, we can also know how to dismantle them. But don't expect the system profiting from perpetual illness to lead the charge.

"Holistic Medicine" Is an Oxymoron

Hopefully, it's becoming more obvious why traditionally educated medical doctors have difficulty practicing natural healthcare. MDs have extensive training, but their education is rooted in disease management, not health creation. It can be done. But it takes humility and a willingness to unlearn deeply ingrained assumptions.

Many MDs who leave Medicine turn to Functional Medicine. But even this can fall into the same trap: swapping drugs for supplements without addressing the root cause. True health isn't about substitution. It's about removing interference. The paradigm of Medicine is inherently incompatible with vitality. Medicine is not broken. It's simply the wrong system for building health, longevity, and vitality. And building vitality certainly falls outside of the scope of "Medicine" and most services coerced by traditional insurance.

The Hidden Hand: How Insurance Dictates Care

Insurance is marketed as a safety net. In reality, it functions more like a gatekeeper. It decides which doctors you can see, what treatments are approved, and how long care should last. This is not about supporting clinical decision-making. It is about controlling cost and protecting profit.

Simply consider that in most conventional clinics, care begins with a question that has nothing to do with your health: "What insurance do you have?" That answer determines which providers you can access, which diagnostics are allowed, and which therapies will be reimbursed. Your entire care plan is shaped by financial contracts, not clinical outcomes.

The issue goes beyond limited coverage. It is embedded in how the system is structured. Reimbursement is tied to short-term symptom control, not long-term health restoration.[45] According to Medicare's own guidelines, "We do not cover services that seek to prevent disease, promote health, or enhance quality of life." That is not a misinterpretation. That is official policy. And Medicare's guidelines set the standard for all other payers.[46]

In other words, care designed to improve health or prevent disease is often denied. But care that fits the disease-management model (i.e., drug therapy or surgical intervention) is covered without resistance. This has created a split system. If you follow the insurance model, your care is built around billing codes and protocols. If you step outside of it, you regain freedom, but you pay out of pocket for that autonomy.

Insurance companies are not accountable to your health. They are accountable to shareholders. Their legal obligation is to reduce costs and increase revenue, even if it means limiting access to care.

This becomes critical when choosing a provider. Because most people do not choose based on trust or outcomes. They choose based on who is "in network." But network status is not a measure of quality. It is a contract between the provider and the insurance company. It tells you who agreed to the terms, not who delivers the best results.

Choosing your doctor based on network status may seem practical. But when the system excludes prevention, rewards quick fixes, and restricts your choices, it is not just unwise. It is dangerous.

The Resistance to the Exodus

What comes next is inevitable. The decline of allopathic dominance is an approaching reality. As patients take control of their own health, the system that profits from keeping them sick will struggle to maintain its authority. The housecleaning has begun, and there will be no return to the unquestioned reign of the white coat. Conventional Medicine will either evolve to recognize vitalism or crumble under the weight of its own failures.

But modern Medicine has a high stake in keeping this story alive. The entire system of diagnosing a disease and prescribing a fix depends on maintaining the belief that disease is something external, something that happens to us. But what if that's not the full story? What if the way we define disease is actually shaping the way we experience it? In the next chapter, we're going to dismantle one of the biggest assumptions in modern Medicine: the germ theory.

CHAPTER 3

The Germ Fallacy

If I could live my life over again, I would devote it to proving that germs seek their natural habitat—diseased tissue—rather than being the cause of dead tissue. In other words, mosquitoes seek the stagnant water, but do not cause the pool to become stagnant.
—Dr. Rudolph Virchow, the "Father of Modern Pathology"

Rethinking What We "Know" About Sickness

Imagine sitting on a crowded airplane. The person next to you begins coughing uncontrollably, and you feel that creeping fear rise: What if I catch it? This deeply ingrained fear of germs defines how we think about sickness and health. It shapes our decisions: washing hands obsessively, wiping down shopping carts, and carrying hand sanitizer like a shield against an invisible enemy.

We've been taught to see illness as an external attack, a battle to be fought against an invisible enemy with pharmaceutical drugs, vaccines, disinfectants, and isolation. But is this fear justified? What if illness is not an invader to be feared but a vital process? What if sickness serves as a purge of toxins and a reset for the body's internal balance and greater adaptability?

The germ theory of disease, developed in the nineteenth century and popularized by Louis Pasteur, claims that microorganisms like bacteria and viruses are the primary cause of illness. According to this theory, these "germs" invade the body from the outside, multiply, and disrupt normal function, resulting in disease. It's a simple and compelling narrative that forms the backbone of Medicine. For over a century, the war on germs has dictated medical interventions. Antibiotics, vaccines, disinfectants, and isolation are used almost entirely based on the assumption that microbes are the primary cause of disease.[1] But what if germs are not the true enemy? What if they are merely opportunistic responders to a preexisting imbalance?

Terrain Theory: The Body as a Garden

Long before Pasteur's germ theory took hold, the dominant model of disease was terrain theory. Terrain theory is the idea that the body's internal environment determines whether disease takes root. Think of your body like a garden. If the soil is rich and healthy, plants thrive, and pests struggle to take hold. But if the soil is depleted and stagnant, fungus, pests, and disease begin to flourish.

Claude Bernard, a contemporary of Pasteur, argued that a weakened terrain invites germs not because they are predators, but because they are scavengers responding to decay. He famously stated:

The microbe is nothing. The terrain is everything.[2]

This means that germs don't "cause" disease in a healthy body, they take advantage of conditions that already favor disease. Rather than signs of failure, symptoms are evidence that the body is actively restoring balance. A fever, for example, isn't something to suppress. It's a sign the body is purging toxins and restoring balance.[3] Coughing and sneezing aren't signs of a problem, they're mechanisms for the body to eliminate waste. When we view illness through the lens of terrain theory, symptoms are evidence of the body's wisdom, not its failure.

This also explains why people can be exposed to the same pathogen, yet some fall ill while others remain healthy. If germs were truly the sole cause of disease, exposure alone would always result in infection. But it doesn't, because the determining factor isn't just the germ, it's the terrain.

Toxins and Disease—A Vitalistic Perspective

But terrain theory isn't complete without discussing toxins. Before germ theory, it was understood that illness was caused by a breakdown of biological material due to toxicity and stagnation (zymotic theory of disease). Physicians observed that outbreaks of illness often followed environmental toxicity: polluted water, rotting food, and poor sanitation.[4] They understood that disease flourished when the body's internal environment became toxic and stagnant. Germs weren't the primary cause; they were recognized as the cleanup crew. We see this today in the way environmental toxins can trigger symptoms virtually identical to those attributed to viruses.

Modern studies confirm that **toxins can produce flu-like symptoms even in the absence of viral exposure**:

- Nurses inhaling pyrethrum-based insecticides experienced sneezing, congestion, and fatigue within hours, symptoms identical to what is called a "viral infection."[5]
- Experiments introducing harmless irritants (saline, beef broth, egg yolk suspensions) into nasal passages triggered congestion, sneezing, and other "flu-like" symptoms.[6]
- Individuals exposed to mold and air pollution report chronic fatigue, sinus congestion, and inflammation: again, symptoms indistinguishable from viral illness.[7]

The takeaway? Toxins, whether from food, chemicals, or stress, trigger the body's cleansing process, which we often mistakenly label as "illness." The body does not become sick from exposure alone, it responds to stressors based on its capacity to maintain balance. While environmental toxins can contribute to nervous system interference, they are not the sole cause of illness. The body is always working to adapt, process, and eliminate what doesn't belong. The key difference between health and sickness isn't whether someone encounters toxins, but whether their body has the capacity to respond effectively.

Imagine two people exposed to the same chemical irritant. One experiences congestion and fatigue, while the other feels nothing. The difference isn't the exposure, it's their internal ability to respond. When the body reaches a threshold of overload, whether from toxic exposure, emotional stress, or nutritional depletion, it activates cleansing mechanisms. We label these processes as "illness," but in reality, they are the body's attempts to purge and restore equilibrium. Rather than seeing toxins as the cause of disease, we should recognize that toxins create interference that the body is constantly working to correct. The real question isn't, "What pathogen made me sick?" but rather, "What is disrupting my body's ability to maintain health?"

Now picture a trampoline park, a place where kids chug fluoride-laced tap water, breathe in off-gassed plastics, are exposed to chemically treated surfaces, and snack on ultra-processed sugar bombs. A few days later, they develop a fever and congestion. The parents might believe that their child "picked something up" at the park but what's the *real* cause? Germs? Or the body's attempt to flush out accumulated toxins?

Germs as Scavengers

If terrain determines health, then germs act as scavengers rather than attackers. Think of a fire. The smoke isn't the cause of the blaze; it's a by-product of something deeper. Likewise, germs don't initiate disease, they respond to imbalanced, devitalized conditions. Just like:

- Vultures don't kill animals, they arrive after death.
- Flies don't cause rotting fruit, they show up because it's already decaying.

The same applies to bacteria and viruses. They appear when conditions in the body invite them. They respond to imbalance and decay. When the body becomes devitalized, germs thrive. Medicine obsesses over eliminating the vultures while ignoring what killed the animal that attracted the vultures in the first place. This is like leaving a rotten banana on the countertop while setting traps for the fruit flies.

Viruses Aren't Alive

If bacteria act as scavengers, responding to weakened terrain, then what about viruses? We've been taught to fear them even more as if they are silent, invisible invaders hijacking our cells and spreading disease. But that understanding couldn't be further from the truth.

Nearly everyone has a skewed understanding of viruses. Most people imagine them as independent, predatory invaders, jumping from person to person like fleas on a dog, spreading sickness wherever they land. But this is a flawed and outdated way of thinking. Unlike bacteria, which are living organisms capable of independent function, viruses are not alive.[8] They don't eat, breathe, or metabolize. They have no agency, no means of movement, and no ability to reproduce on their own.

A virus is nothing more than a strand of genetic material, DNA or RNA, encased in a protein shell. It cannot "infect" in the way we've been led to believe. It does not actively seek out hosts, nor does it "attack" the body. Instead, viruses are triggered within us, often as a response to toxicity, stress, or a necessary biological adaptation.[9] The body produces and utilizes viral particles for internal communication, cellular repair, and even genetic upgrades.

This is why sickness, especially in children, is often followed by a leap in development: a clearer mind, a growth spurt, or newfound skills.[10] What we call "illness" may, in fact, be a recalibration, a purge, a healing event rather than an attack. The body isn't at war. It's intelligently responding to its environment in a way that has sustained human life for millennia.

Can You "Catch" Sickness?

If viruses don't function like predators, then why do so many people assume sickness spreads like wildfire? Why does it seem like colds, flus, and other illnesses move through families, workplaces, and schools? The answer is not what we've been led to believe.

Medicine attributes the common cold and influenza to contagious viruses, with scientists asserting that these viruses are transmitted through one of three primary methods: droplets, aerosols, or contact with contaminated surfaces. But the scientific evidence supporting this claim is surprisingly weak. A 2003 literature review found no published studies providing evidence of human-to-human transmission.[11] Similarly, a later study on influenza concluded that the illness does not spread through the typical sick-to-well transmission model.[12] These findings challenge everything we assume about viral contagion.

During the COVID-19 pandemic, public health officials implemented widespread mask mandates, believing that blocking droplets would stop the spread. Yet, in cities with the strictest mask mandates and social distancing enforcement, the death rates were actually higher than in cities without them.[13] If the germ theory were accurate, the death rates should have been the lowest. That's because exposure to germs is not the predictive factor of whether you will become "sick."

Systematic reviews on the subject often conclude that airborne transmission plays a minimal role, if any, in spreading respiratory illnesses, and there is no solid evidence linking large respiratory droplets to disease transmission.[14] Several reviews have further highlighted the difficulty in demonstrating aerosol transmission for well-studied pathogens like SARS-CoV-1 and SARS-CoV-2. Scientists have failed to produce direct evidence proving that viruses spread through the air or by touch.

Dr. Rodermond's Experiments

For over a century, the assumption that sickness spreads through germs has gone largely unchallenged. But history tells a different story. If contagious diseases really operated as we've been told, shouldn't we find clear, consistent proof? Instead, when skeptics have tested the theory in real-world conditions, the results have been anything but predictable. One such doctor was Matthew Rodermund, a Wisconsin physician in the early 1900s.[15] Dr. Rodermund was no stranger to the contagion controversy. Determined to challenge the prevailing belief that smallpox was highly contagious through direct contact, he performed a bold and shocking experiment. Entering the room of a young girl with smallpox, he first asked her mother if she feared contracting the disease. When she said no, Rodermund began bursting the girl's blisters and smearing the pus onto his own face, beard, hands, and clothing.

For the next forty-eight hours, Dr. Rodermund went about his life without washing or changing. He ate dinner with his family, consulted patients, and played cards at the local Businessman's Club, where, by his own account, he touched the faces and hands of at least ten people. The following day, he traveled to a nearby town, consulted with twenty-seven more patients, and continued his routine as though nothing unusual had occurred. No one around him contracted smallpox.

Dr. Rodermund was adamant that smallpox was not contagious. Over a span of fifteen years, he repeated this experiment more than a dozen times, always with the same result.[16] His actions infuriated public health officials, who quarantined him. Undeterred, Rodermund broke quarantine, traveling to multiple cities to continue his demonstrations. His defiance ultimately led to his arrest, sparking widespread public outrage and heated debates about the true nature of disease transmission.

While Rodermund's experiment was extreme and controversial, it forces us to ask an uncomfortable question: If exposure alone causes disease, why didn't he or those around him become ill?

The answer is simple: Exposure alone is not the deciding factor. The body's current state of resilience determines if a purge or cleanse is necessary. Rodermund didn't "defy" germ theory, he proved that the body's internal condition is the determining factor.

Outbreaks in Isolation

If sickness were truly about germs jumping from person to person, then outbreaks should never happen in places where no outside germs can enter. Yet history is filled with cases that defy this expectation. The germ theory, which asserts that diseases like influenza are caused by contagious viruses spreading from person to person within a seven-day window of contagion, unravels when examined in the context of isolated outbreaks. According to the medical model, viruses like influenza are thought to be contagious for about a day before symptoms appear and up to seven days afterward. However, history provides numerous examples of outbreaks in isolated settings that defy this explanation.

The "Antarctic Anomalies" of 1969 presents a baffling example.[17] Researchers and workers stationed in Antarctica, completely cut off from the outside world for months, experienced an outbreak of influenza-like illness. With no newcomers to introduce a virus and no contact with the global population, this raises the question: could something other than contagion be at play?

In 2020, doctors reported COVID-like illnesses in remote communities with no known contact with infected individuals, defying standard contagion models.[18] These cases highlight a critical flaw in the germ-centric model: it cannot account for illnesses arising in isolated groups. Instead, it highlights that the roots of sickness are not external invaders but internal conditions shaped by shared environments, stressors, and terrain.

Exposure to Viruses and Bacteria: Nature's Genetic Upgrade

Far from being passive victims of germs, our bodies use viral and bacterial exposure as an opportunity to adapt, strengthening our genetic resilience over time.[19] Our bodies are equipped with an intricate system that thrives on interaction with the world around us. When we are exposed to viruses and bacteria, these encounters equip and enhance our immune system. Like a skilled coach pushing an athlete to grow stronger, microorganisms provide the stimulus our bodies need to adapt. This process acts as a kind of genetic upgrade, refining our DNA and epigenetically programming our bodies for resilience and future challenges.

Viruses and bacteria serve as teachers, introducing our immune system to new challenges. These microorganisms expose our bodies to tiny pieces of their structure that the immune system can recognize, called antigens. When the immune system encounters these antigens, it mounts a response, creating specialized cells, such as memory T cells and B cells, which "remember" the invader. This memory equips the body to respond more effectively if the pathogen is encountered again.

The body's response to viral and bacterial exposure is also facilitated by exosomes.[20] These tiny extracellular vesicles are released by cells under stress or during an immune response. Exosomes act as messengers, carrying genetic material, proteins, and signaling molecules to other cells. They orchestrate a coordinated response, ensuring that the body adapts efficiently.

But the relationship goes deeper than immune training. Viruses, in particular, can integrate their genetic material into our DNA. While this might sound alarming, this process, known as horizontal gene transfer, has played a pivotal role in human adaptation over time. Viral DNA doesn't just linger in our genome; it can become part of the blueprint that makes us who we are.[21]

Viruses and Cancer

Emerging research suggests that certain viral infections may play a role in reducing the risk of developing specific types of cancer. For instance, a study published in *BMC Medicine* found that individuals with a history of herpes zoster (shingles) had a decreased risk of developing low-grade glioma, a type of brain tumor.[22]

Additionally, recent studies have observed that severe COVID-19 infections can lead to tumor regression. Researchers at Northwestern Medicine Canning Thoracic Institute discovered that the RNA from the SARS-CoV-2 virus can stimulate the development of a unique subset of immune cells, termed "inducible nonclassical monocytes" (I-NCMs).[23] These cells have demonstrated the ability to infiltrate tumors and directly attack cancer cells, resulting in tumor shrinkage. This effect has been noted in cancers such as melanoma, lung, breast, and colorectal. These findings suggest that certain viral exposures might stimulate the immune system in ways that confer protective effects against specific cancers.

Notably, the measles virus has been investigated for its oncolytic properties, the ability to selectively infect and destroy cancer cells. A remarkable case reported by the Mayo Clinic involved a patient with multiple myeloma, an incurable bone marrow cancer, who achieved complete remission for six months following treatment with a high dose of a modified measles germ virus.[24]

Research has indicated an association between a history of chickenpox infection and a reduced risk of developing certain types of brain tumors. A study conducted by the University of California, San Francisco, found that individuals who had experienced chickenpox had a lower incidence of gliomas compared to those who had not.[25]

This shows that when the body mediates infection, it upgrades on a cellular level, leaving it more resilient and adaptable for future exposures and aging. Think of your immune system as a sophisticated software program. Viruses and bacteria act like updates, patching vulnerabilities and adding new features. Each exposure enhances the immune system's database, allowing it to recognize a broader range of threats. This proactive preparation not only strengthens your defenses against that specific pathogen but also equips your immune system to handle similar challenges in the future.

This phenomenon is why children who experience common illnesses, like measles or chickenpox, often emerge with stronger, more adaptable immune systems. Studies suggest that individuals who contract these illnesses in childhood may have a lower risk of developing certain cancers and chronic diseases later in life.[26] The immune system isn't just fighting off invaders. It's designed to use these exposures to adapt and evolve.

Germ Theory versus Terrain Theory

Bacteria and viruses don't behave the way we've been taught. They don't act like tiny assassins floating around, hunting for victims. They emerge in response to the state of the host. They express, change form, or multiply based on the condition of the host. They are shaped by their environment.

So what about using a virus to kill cancer?

That does not contradict terrain theory. It actually reinforces it.

When the terrain of a tumor becomes toxic and oxygen-deprived, it creates an environment where certain microbes thrive. Some of these microbes can help break down dying or abnormal tissue. In modern Medicine, certain viruses are introduced on purpose to accelerate this process. They do not cure cancer, but they can help the body clear something it was struggling to clean up on its own.

It's an example of a "trigger" for a cleanup response.

Bottom line:

Germs are not the cause. They are the result.

If you want true healing, you have to address the imbalanced terrain and stop waging war on the cleanup crew.

The Forest's Network: A Model for Human Vitalism

Our bodies don't operate in isolation. Just as viruses play a role in enhancing biological resilience, the entire natural world thrives on interconnected signals. Nowhere is this more evident than in forests. Forests provide an extraordinary example of interconnectedness through a network sometimes called the "wood wide web."[27] Beneath the soil, fungi form vast networks that connect the roots of trees, allowing them to communicate and share resources. When one tree is under attack, say, from harmful fungi or pests, it sends chemical signals through this network to warn others. Neighboring trees respond by bolstering their defenses, producing protective compounds or redirecting resources to strengthen their resilience.

These protective defenses might appear as negative. For instance, a tree threatened by pests might release compounds that repel the invaders but also cause leaves to discolor or drop prematurely. To an uninformed observer, this might seem like a sign of decline rather than a deliberate act of self-preservation.

Now imagine applying the germ-combating approach to the forest. A scientist observes these defenses, such as leaf discoloration, fungi on the roots, or chemical secretions, and interprets them as symptoms of invasion to be eradicated. The scientist might propose removing the affected trees (quarantine), spraying fungicides (disinfectants), or sterilizing the soil (antibiotics). But what would the result be? The removal of these defenses would disrupt the forest's natural balance, leaving it more vulnerable to future threats.

This mirrors how we often treat our bodies. Symptoms like fever, coughing, or vomiting are viewed as malfunctions to suppress, rather than as evidence of the body's intelligent efforts to restore balance and protect itself. Just as the forest thrives through its interconnected network, our bodies depend on complex systems of adaptation and communication. By misunderstanding these processes, we risk harming the very systems that sustain life.

From a vitalistic perspective, the "virus" might actually be necessary for cellular adaptation. The exposure to microorganisms might not be about "catching" a virus but about receiving a biological message, a set of instructions for upgrading and adapting the body.

Just as trees in a forest respond collectively to environmental stressors, human bodies operate in synchrony with those around them. Our biology is not isolated; it is constantly adapting to shared signals, whether they come from the environment, emotions, or even other people. One striking example of this interconnectedness is found in the phenomenon of menstrual synchrony.

Menstrual Synchrony: Alignment through Shared Signals

Studies have documented that women who live together or spend significant time in close proximity more often than not experience their cycles falling into rhythm. This phenomenon, referred to as the "McClintock Effect," is not due to hormonal "contagion" but rather an innate biological response to shared environments and energetic fields.[28]

From a vitalistic perspective, this synchrony is evidence of the body's intelligence, operating in harmony with natural rhythms. These shared patterns serve a purpose, such as promoting social cohesion or enhancing group survival. In ancient communities, synchronized cycles may have maximized opportunities for reproduction and collective care of offspring.

Similarly, what we interpret as the "spread" of illness might not be the transmission of germs but the synchronization of bodies responding to shared conditions. When a family or community experiences a common stressor, be it a seasonal shift, a toxin in the environment, or emotional upheaval, their bodies will align in a collective detoxification process. This vitalistic understanding reframes "contagion" as an adaptive, communal response, mirroring the same principles seen in menstrual synchrony.

Putting It Together: Why Do Families Get Sick Together? A Shared Purge, Not Contagion

At this point, it should be obvious that germs and viruses are not the primary cause for sickness. However, there's one key element that must be addressed to fully understand the concept that germs aren't the cause of sickness or disease: the concept of "passing it around." What if families don't "spread" sickness at all, but instead go through a shared purge, a necessary detoxification in response to common stressors?

For generations, we've been taught that illness is something we "pass around" like a game of microbial hot potato. One child gets sick, then another, then a parent, reinforcing the belief that germs hop from person to person like invisible invaders. But we've been misreading the signals.

Think about it: families breathe the same air, eat the same food, experience the same seasonal shifts, and navigate similar emotional stressors. When one body initiates a detoxification process (fever, congestion, fatigue), others may follow suit. Not because of germ exposure, but because their systems are responding to the same underlying stressors.

Dr. Zach Bush explains this process on a broader scale:[29]

> *Viruses are not pathogens that can leap out of nowhere and attack us, but they are the mechanism for genetically transferring information between species.*

"Expressing Health"

Imagine eating a pound of E. coli–contaminated food and your body didn't vomit. That would be alarming. It would be a clear sign your system wasn't responding appropriately.

The act of vomiting is not a failure; it's evidence of a healthy response to an extreme toxin.[30] A fever burns off pathogens. A runny nose flushes irritants. A cough clears the airways. Each of these is a deliberate, intelligent action initiated by your body to protect and heal itself. In our family, we don't say, "Little Johnnie is sick." We say, "He's expressing health." Because that's exactly what's happening. What we call "illness" is often the body *expressing health*: purging toxins, recalibrating systems, and restoring balance.

This flips the entire script: health isn't about avoiding exposure; it's about embracing the body's natural processes of renewal. Just like the trees in a forest, human bodies communicate and respond collectively within shared environments.

Instead of saying, "We're passing it around," consider:

- "Our bodies are recalibrating."
- "We're moving through a natural cleanse."
- "This is a necessary detox."

This shift in language is empowerment. Instead of fearing symptoms as proof of weakness, we recognize them as evidence of vitality in action. Next time a cold moves through your household or classroom, ask, "What common stressors have we all been exposed to?" You might be surprised how often a so-called "illness" follows the introduction of a new toxic cleaner, a wave of emotional stress, or dietary shifts. The body doesn't break down randomly; it intelligently adapts. By shifting how we talk about illness, we move from fear to empowerment, from suppression to trust.

To see symptoms as failures is to misunderstand the brilliance of your design. Illness is not the breakdown of health but the recalibration of it. Recognizing this truth shifts the narrative: health is not about the absence of symptoms but about the body's ability to respond with vitality, balance, and precision.

The Expectation Effect: How Beliefs Shape Illness

No discussion of germs and illness is complete without addressing what may be the most overlooked variable of all—the mind. Germ theory treats the body as a machine and germs as invaders, but it leaves out the one system that can influence every other: your thoughts. The Expectation Effect is a powerful example.

A 2020 study found that people who anticipated getting the flu were far more likely to report symptoms.[31] In other words, fear and belief can become a self-fulfilling prophecy.

This is not new. During the Spanish flu pandemic, Chicago's public health director warned, "Worry kills more than the disease."[32] Fear amplifies symptoms and weakens recovery, while positive states like optimism and purpose have been shown to protect against colds and flu, even under the same viral exposure.[33]

Society's fixation on germs,

A Real-Life Example:
Rob used to immediately suppress every sniffle and headache with over-the-counter meds. After learning about the body's design, he started listening instead of fighting. When a fever hit, he rested, hydrated with water, and trusted his body. He prioritized the health of his nervous system. Over time, recovery became faster, and he noticed fewer illnesses altogether. Rob realized resilience wasn't in fighting symptoms—it was in fortifying his mind and body. He also lost one hundred pounds, reversed type 2 diabetes, and got off all his blood pressure and cholesterol medications. Those are simply side effects of living vitalistically.

outbreaks, and illness primes us for sickness. But the same mental pathways can be redirected. By replacing fear of sickness with trust in the
body's intelligent responses, we can shift from being primed for vulner-
ability to being fortified for health.

Fear of contagion is one of the most powerful forces in Medicine. It
triggers quick decisions and shuts down critical thinking.[34] By now, you've
seen the cracks in the germ theory. But those cracks run deeper than you
think. Foundational medical protocols have been built on the idea that
germs must be stopped at all costs. The vaccine program is one of those.
Healthy children face almost no serious risk from these so-called preventable diseases. But still, "vaccines save lives" is one of the most deeply
rooted beliefs in medicine today.

In the next chapter, we examine the vaccine decision for what it truly
is, a decision. One that deserves clarity about what's in vaccines, whether
they are necessary, and the impact they may have on your health.

CHAPTER 4

The Vaccine Decision:
The Ingredients, the Evidence,
and the Impact

Any possible doubts, whether or not well founded, about the safety of the vaccine cannot be allowed to exist in view of the need to assure that the vaccine will continue to be used to the maximum extent consistent with the nation's public health objectives.
— Federal Register, vol. 49, no 107 (June 1, 1984): 23007

Informed Consent in an Era of Medical Mandates

"Informed consent" is the cornerstone of ethical medicine, yet in the world of vaccines that principle has quietly eroded. Parents are told that children must receive state-mandated shots to attend school or participate in summer camps; healthcare workers are told they must receive shots to get or keep employment; pregnant women are told they need shots or they will endanger their baby. By definition, this is a breach of informed consent because the decision is coerced.[1] Ethically, people must know the benefits and risks of an intervention, the alternatives, and what happens if they do nothing, and then be free to decide without any element of force.

I have helped too many families who were dismissed from their pediatrician's office simply for asking questions about "required" vaccines. When asking for more information is treated as dangerous, the freedom to make your own health decisions is stifled. If you cannot say no, it is not a choice; it is "informed coercion." As a self-reliant, responsible parent, you must make health decisions that reflect your convictions and your family's best interests. Outsourcing the care of ourselves and our children to experts has not served our health or our freedom.

This is not speculation. At the October 2024 ACIP meeting, members discussed how wording affects compliance.[2] ACIP stands for Advisory Committee on Immunization Practices and is the CDC's group of experts that puts shots on the shot schedule. In ACIP guidance, shots are either universally recommended or they are recommended for "shared clinical decision making" where the patient and the doctor should decide based on individual risk factors whether the intervention is appropriate. Almost all shots on the schedule are universally recommended by ACIP.

During the meeting, several members said "shared clinical decision making" "doesn't work" for their goal because fewer people will say yes. The committee emphasized that telling people they *should* get a shot yields more compliance than saying they *may*. In that framework, decisions based on individual risk, made between a doctor and a patient, are treated as an obstacle to the policy objective of universal vaccination.

To reclaim our children's health and our right to make medical decisions, we must learn how to make the vaccine decision intentionally, critically, and with all the information necessary. That begins with understanding four vital questions:

1. Why do these products exist, and are they truly needed?
2. Why did the childhood vaccine schedule explode in the late 1990s?
3. What's actually in the products?
4. What are the real-world fallouts in American health that coincide with the vaccine schedule?

The Premise of the Program: "Vaccines Are the Greatest Gift to Public Health"—or Are They?

This is the message we've been sold: that vaccines are the bedrock of modern health, a miraculous shield against disease and the foundation of national security. But when we pause and look beyond the narrative and beyond American borders, the cracks in that perspective begin to show.

Consider Japan, a developed country of 127 million people, with some of the healthiest children in the world[3] and the highest "healthy life expectancy."[4] Japan also uses a comparatively less intensive childhood vaccination schedule by number of shots and visit frequency, and there is no blanket mandate; vaccines are routinely recommended rather than compulsory (required by law). The United States, by contrast, follows one of the most intensive schedules, beginning in pregnancy and at birth with hepatitis B, with 72+ doses recommended by age eighteen.[5] Yet American children fare worse. We have the highest infant mortality rate[6] (children dying before their first birthday) of any industrialized country and sky-rocketing rates of chronic illness in children (daily suffering and a reduced quality of life).[7]

The country with the most vaccines also has the sickest kids. If vaccines were the key to long life and robust childhood health, wouldn't American children be leading the pack? If this is medical advancement, why are our children falling apart behaviorally, emotionally, and physically? Is the per-ceived benefit of reduced childhood infections like measles, mumps, and chickenpox worth the unintended effects of population-wide overvaccina-tion? That might seem like a bold statement, but I haven't met a person yet who looks at the current childhood vaccine schedule for American children and isn't concerned about the sheer number of doses and their timing.

How can anyone truly know if the vaccine program and the CDC's recommendations have done more harm than good when according to the Institute of Medicine the childhood vaccine schedule has not been studied.[8]

No studies have compared the differences in health outcomes that some stakeholders questioned between entirely unimmunized popu-lations of children and fully immunized children . . . existing research has not been designed to test the entire immunization schedule. Studies designed to examine the long-term effects of the cumulative number of vaccines or other aspects of the immunization schedule

HEALTH FREEDOM INSTITUTE
The CDC's Childhood Vaccine Schedule
May 2025

1962
OPV
Smallpox
DTP

5 DOSES

healthfreedominstitute.com

1983
DTP (2 months)
OPV (2 months)
DTP (4 months)
OPV (4 months)
DTP (6 months)
MMR (15 months)
DTP (18 months)
OPV (18 months)
DTP (4 years)
OPV (4 years)
Td (15 years)

24 DOSES

2025
Influenza (pregnancy)
RSV (pregnancy)
Tdap (pregnancy)
Hep B (birth)
Hep B (2 months)
Rotavirus (2 months)
DTaP (2 months)
HIB (2 months)
PCV (2 months)
IPV (2 months)
Rotavirus (4 months)
DTaP (4 months)
HIB (4 months)
PCV (4 months)
IPV (4 months)
Hep B (6 months)
Rotavirus (6 months)
DTaP (6 months)
HIB (6 months)
PCV (6 months)
IPV (6 months)
Influenza (6 months)
Influenza (7 months)
HIB (12 months)
PCV (12 months)
MMR (12 months)
Varicella (12 months)
Hep A (12 months)
DTaP (15 months)
Influenza (18 months)
Hep A (18 months)

Influenza (2 years)
Influenza (3 years)
DTaP (4 years)
IPV (4 years)
MMR (4 years)
Varicella (4 years)
Influenza (4 years)
Influenza (5 years)
Influenza (6 years)
Influenza (7 years)
Influenza (8 years)
Influenza (9 years)
Influenza (10 years)
Influenza (11 years)
Meningococcal (11 years)
HPV x3 (9-15 years)
Influenza (12 years)
Influenza (13 years)
Influenza (14 years)
Influenza (15 years)
Influenza (16 years)
Meningococcal (16 years)
Influenza (17 years)

72 DOSES
before age 18

(Children who miss shots, travel internationally, are high risk, immunocompromised, have special medical indications will get more. Doses counted by earliest age and max doses recommended.)

Since 1986, Pharma has not been liable for vaccine injury or death.

- Lawsuits from vaccines like polio and DTaP were putting manufacturers out of business.
- In 1986, Congress passed the National Childhood Vaccine Injury Act so pharma could no longer be sued for vaccine injury or death.
- The US Supreme Court decided in 2011 manufacturers also can't be sued for design defects.
- The 1986 Act created a special vaccine court where over $5.3 billion dollars in injuries have been paid out for vaccine injuries to children or their families, only a fraction of the claims.
- After the protections of the normal court process were removed, the government-recommended vaccine schedule exploded, and increases every year.
- Since 1986, there has been an estimated fourfold increase in chronic disease for American children.
- The most compensated claim for injury is from the annual influenza vaccine, however HPV is proportionately the most.
- The CDC's schedule is not law, but many states look to it to create their own vaccine mandates for childhood education and many adopt it fully, making federal guidance into state law.
- What about COVID? Over 1 million adverse events were reported for COVID shots alone since the first EUA in December 2020. One shot doubled the entire database in 2 years. It can take longer than 2 years for vaccine injury to show itself.
  - In May 2025, HHS did away with COVID shot recommendations for healthy children and pregnant women.

healthfreedominstitute.com

have not been conducted. Key elements of the entire schedule—the number, frequency, timing, order, and age at administration of vaccines—have not been systematically examined in research studies.

—2013 IOM Report: The Childhood Immunization Schedule and Safety: Stakeholder Concerns, Scientific Evidence, and Future Studies

Why Did Vaccine-Preventable Diseases Decline?

Many assume vaccines are responsible for the dramatic decline in infectious disease rates and deaths throughout the 1900s. Is that a belief or is that knowledge based in fact? The greatest improvements in public health—declines in deaths from diseases like measles, diphtheria, and scarlet fever—occurred *before* vaccines were introduced and well before they were mandated for school. See for example figure 19 below showing the measles death rates falling prior to 1963, the year that the first measles vaccines were licensed.[9]

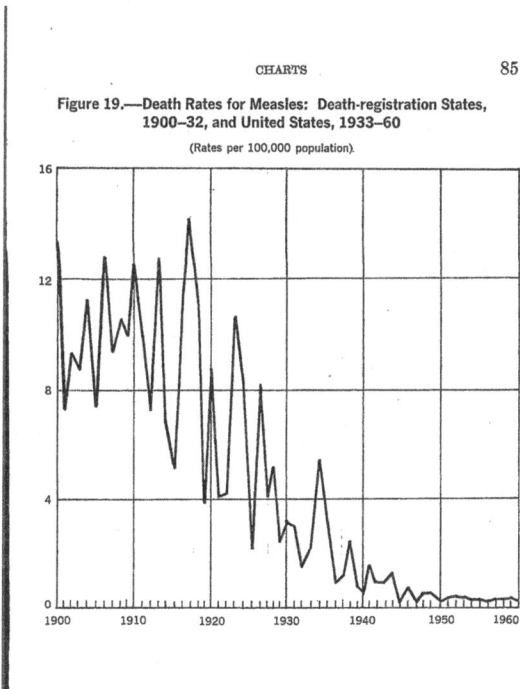

CHARTS 85

Figure 19.—Death Rates for Measles: Death-registration States, 1900–32, and United States, 1933–60

(Rates per 100,000 population).

Figure 19: Death Rates for Measles: Death-registration States, 1900–32, and United States, 1933–60 https://www.cdc.gov/nchs/data/vsus/vsrates1940_60.pdf.

According to epidemiologists from Johns Hopkins and the CDC, nearly 90 percent of the decline in infectious disease mortality among children occurred before 1940, before vaccines or antibiotics were widely used.[10] We didn't vaccinate our way out of sickness. We cleaned up our water, our food, and our living. Public health won that battle. Pharma took the credit.

Polio, often cited as the ultimate vaccine success story, illustrates the deeper truth: Medicine didn't so much eliminate the disease as redefine it. Prior to the vaccine rollout in 1955, "polio" referred to a broad spectrum of symptoms, including acute flaccid paralysis, muscular weakness, even stomach viruses. The diagnosis was based largely on observation, not lab confirmation. After the introduction of the vaccine, the criteria for diagnosing paralytic polio changed drastically. A case that would have been counted as paralytic polio in 1954 now had to involve paralysis lasting at least sixty days to qualify. As statistician Dr. Bernard Greenberg testified to Congress, this semantic shift alone reduced reported polio cases, not the vaccine.[11]

Figure 5. Polio cases were predetermined to decrease when the medical definition of polio was changed

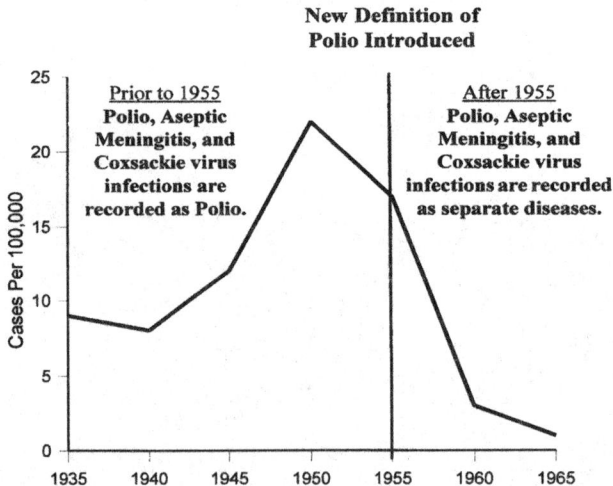

Source: Congressional Hearings, May 1962; and National Morbidity Reports taken from U.S. Public Health surveillance reports.

Figure 5: New Definition of Polio Introduced

The Decline of Polio . . . or Just a Name Change?

Beginning in the mid-1990s, the global health community declared victory over polio, thanks to aggressive vaccination campaigns, especially in countries like India. Wild poliovirus cases dropped significantly. But here's what few people noticed.

At the same time wild polio was declining, cases of Acute Flaccid Paralysis (AFP), the very condition used to track polio, spiked dramatically (see graphic below). In India, AFP cases rose from about 10,000 in 1996 to over 60,000 per year by 2011.[12] These weren't mild cases. Many of these children were left paralyzed, disabled, or dead, just like traditional polio victims. But because they tested negative for wild poliovirus, they were written off as "non-polio AFP."

If polio had truly been eradicated, one would expect paralysis cases to plummet. Instead, paralysis remained, just under a new name.

Polio out—AFP in?

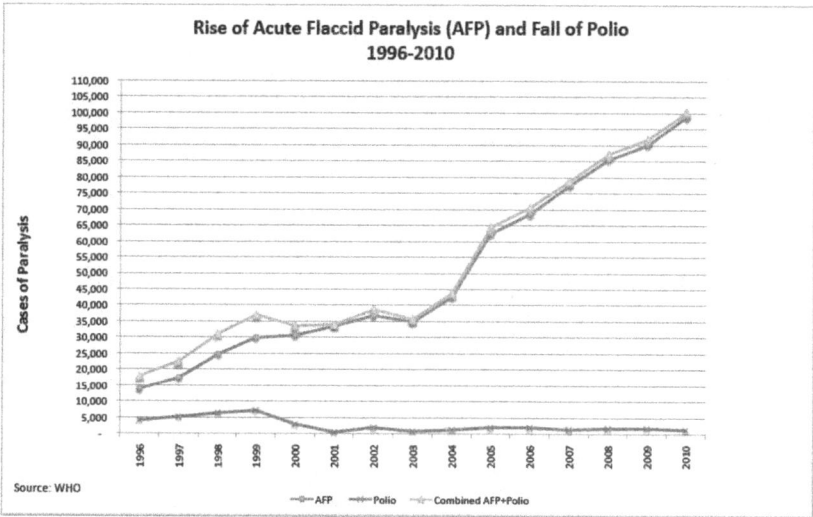

Rise of Acute Flaccid Paralysis and Fall of Polio 1996–2010.

Polio by Another Name?

AFP isn't a statistical outlier. It's one example of the semantic reclassification that began decades earlier. Before 1954, the diagnosis of "poliomyelitis" could include a wide range of neurological and infectious conditions:

- Transverse myelitis
- Viral or "aseptic" meningitis
- Gullain-Barre syndrome
- Endemic cholera
- Spinal meningitis
- Spinal apoplexy
- Acute flaccid paralysis

In other words, many forms of paralysis and neurological inflammation were routinely diagnosed as "polio." But as the vaccine era gained momentum, the diagnostic criteria narrowed, and those same conditions were now given different names.

This shift allowed the appearance of progress, even if the number of paralyzed children remained the same or worse.

Could the Polio Vaccine Itself Be Driving AFP?

A growing number of researchers have asked a hard question: could the vaccine itself be contributing to this rise in non-polio AFP?

Multiple studies, including those published in *The Lancet Infectious Diseases* and *Indian Pediatrics*, have documented a dose-dependent relationship between the number of oral polio vaccine (OPV) doses and the incidence of non-polio AFP.[13] Regions receiving the most aggressive vaccination efforts often reported the highest AFP rates.

Some researchers point to possible mechanisms:

- Chronic gut inflammation from repeated OPV exposure
- Disruption of the microbiome
- Vaccine-derived viral shedding
- Heightened susceptibility to other enteroviruses

Even though the cases tested negative for *wild* poliovirus, some may have stemmed from vaccine-derived strains, or resulted from indirect iatrogenic effects of repeated mass immunization.

Incentivized Positive Cases . . . Was COVID a Replay?

We've seen how redefining a disease can create the illusion of progress. But what happens when you financially reward the diagnosis itself? That's exactly what happened with polio.

In the years leading up to the polio vaccine, the National Foundation for Infantile Paralysis offered families lifetime medical care if their child was diagnosed with polio.[14] Not surprisingly, diagnoses surged. Then, almost overnight, diagnostic criteria changed. Conditions once labeled "polio" were renamed. Cases that would have been counted before the vaccine were now excluded. As statistician Dr. Bernard Greenberg explained, "In 1953 we started reporting a new disease."[15]

This wasn't just medical progress. It was a rebranding campaign, fueled by incentives on both sides—first to inflate polio numbers before the vaccine, then to deflate them after.

Fast-forward to 2020. Suddenly, COVID-19 became the diagnosis of choice. Hospitals received higher reimbursements for COVID-positive cases. Deaths *with* COVID were often reported as deaths *from* COVID. PCR tests with high cycle thresholds flooded the data with false positives, inflating case numbers and sustaining fear. Cancer deaths plummeted as COVID deaths soared. The seasonal flu all but vanished, because everything became COVID.

The more cases, the more funding. The more fear, the more compliance. Sound familiar? The playbook didn't just repeat, it was put on steroids.

Hospitals were given financial incentives to diagnose, treat, and report COVID-19 cases. Here's how it worked:[16]

1. 20 percent Bonus: Under the CARES Act, hospitals received an automatic 20 percent increase in Medicare reimbursements for each COVID-positive diagnosis.
2. Positive Test = Payment: To receive the bonus, a PCR test was required. The more people tested—and tested positive—the more money flowed in.
3. Ventilators Tripled the Payout: If a COVID patient was put on a ventilator, hospitals could receive up to $39,000, compared to just $13,000 for standard care.

4. Cause of Death? Assumed. COVID could be listed as the cause of
death without a positive test, so long as it was "assumed" to have
contributed.

Incentivize the diagnosis. Inflate the numbers. Roll out the "solution."
Then redefine the terms to declare victory.

It worked for COVID in the 2020s. And it worked with polio in the
1950s.

What's Really in Vaccines?

Do you know the ingredients in the vaccines that are recommended for
your child? If you don't, it is impossible to make an informed decision, to
understand the risks and benefits. Unfortunately, leading virologists are
either confused or less than transparent about what is actually in a vaccine,
which makes it that much more important to inform yourself.

The CDC does publish the full list of vaccine ingredients, but it can be
difficult to decipher. Vaccines are not just a dose of weakened virus. They
are pharmaceutical products containing aluminum adjuvants (known
neurotoxins), mercury derivatives (like thimerosal), preservatives like
monosodium glutamate (MSG), foreign proteins, fertilizers, heavy metals,
detergents, insect parts, aborted fetal cells, and in some cases, genetically
modified ingredients.[17] You can look up the current CDC Excipient table,
but chances are it will not mean much without decoding that "bovine
albumin" is a protein derived from cow plasma or that "WI-38" is aborted
fetal cells, "Polymyxin B" is an antibiotic or that "2-Phenoxyethanol" is
a chemical preservative, and the list goes on. To be fair, the cocktail of
foreign proteins and chemicals play a part in the function and delivery of
the product. For example, metals act as an "adjuvant" to help offend the
immune system and cause it to react to the proteins in the product; preservatives help the product last from factory to administration; and proteins
are used to host the viruses.

The big caveat is that many vaccines have never been tested against a
true placebo like saline. Instead, they're tested against other vaccines or
aluminum-based solutions, making it nearly impossible to detect the true
rate of adverse events.

We are told vaccines are "safe and effective," yet:

- Routine childhood vaccines are not tested for their effect on fertility. See section 13.1 of the package inserts for the shots.[18]
- No vaccine has been tested for carcinogenic or mutagenic potential. Once again, take a look at section 13.1 of the package inserts.[19]
- Safety follow-up in clinical trials often lasts just a few weeks and the CDC willingly relies upon future post market safety data when making a recommendation for every American schoolchild to receive a shot.
- The full CDC schedule—the one with seventy-two doses—has *never* been tested in its entirety against a completely unvaccinated cohort for intended effects (vaccine preventable disease rates) or unintended effects (chronic disease, sudden death, heart failure, kidney failure etc.).[20]
- According to US law, vaccines belong to a class of products that are "unavoidably unsafe," meaning statutorily that there are some things on the market that cannot be made safe or else they won't be effective.[21]
- US regulations also provide that package inserts for vaccines should include "*only* those adverse events for which there is some basis to believe there is a *causal relationship* between the drug and the occurrence of the adverse event." 21 CFR 201.57.[22] And there are over one hundred serious adverse events listed on the package inserts.[23]
- No routine vaccine was tested for overall effect on mortality before being introduced.

Even worse, the Vaccine Adverse Event Reporting System (VAERS)—the publicly available online database for tracking harm or death post vaccination—is estimated to capture less than 1 percent of all adverse events.[24] In 2018, over 58,000 adverse events were reported, including more than 400 deaths.[25] What would the numbers look like if reporting were enforced and complete? VAERS is the result of the National Childhood Vaccine

Injury Act and is required to be used by providers that administer vaccines or observe a vaccine injury, but there is no enforcement mechanism within the law. So it is greatly underutilized. Once again, crippling informed decision-making, especially for a class of products that has a safety profile which relies heavily on post-market data. Without accurate and available reporting, how can a parent possibly know whether the benefit of a product outweighs its risks? The good news is that there are mountains of information out there, if you go looking for it. This chapter covers the tip of the iceberg to understand the questions that need to be asked and some of the information to be considered.

The Schedule Explosion: What Happened in the Late Nineties?

Up until the 1990s, children received just a handful of vaccines. But that changed dramatically on the heels of a major shift in the vaccine industry: In 1986, Congress passed the National Childhood Vaccine Injury Act ("The 1986 Act"), which granted vaccine manufacturers and clinical providers immunity from liability for vaccine injury or death.[26] This law was the result of years of lobbying by the vaccine manufacturers because lawsuits from post-vaccine injury, most commonly polio and DTaP, were becoming extremely costly. The industry essentially said that it would stop making the government's vaccines for its vaccine program if the Reagan administration did not shield them from the financial risks from injuries in those that use their products.

With no legal or financial consequence for harm, pharmaceutical companies were suddenly free to flood the market with new products—and they did. Not only did companies like Merck and Pfizer get to slash a major line item in their budgets—liability from lawsuits—but federal, state, and local governments also took on another huge budget line item with mandates. Who needs to spend millions in nationwide marketing campaigns when every school and state health department follows the Centers for Disease Control and does it for you? All that to say, the market was ripe for profit in an unmatched way because the new law removed free market forces that force for-profit companies to make safe products.

The 1986 Act also created a special vaccine court where over $5.3 billion dollars in injuries have been paid out for vaccine injuries to children or their families, which only represents a fraction of the claims filed.[27] The grave injustice about the special court is that no discovery is allowed. This means that the injured family cannot request documents, research, and communications from the manufacturer or doctor to find out what information they had or knew about the child's exposure to harm. This keeps the public in a chronic cycle of closed-circuit communications where the government-sponsored, industry narrative shapes the cultural understanding of the vaccine program.

By the late 1990s, the schedule had exploded and continues to increase year after year.[28] New vaccines were added for chickenpox, rotavirus, pneumococcal disease, hepatitis A and B, influenza, and more. Today's infants receive more than twenty-six antigens—foreign substances that stimulate an immune response—by their first birthday.[29] The CDC recommends seventy-two doses by the time a child turns eighteen.

Yet, despite this explosion in vaccine delivery, American children have become sicker, not healthier. There has been an estimated fourfold increase in chronic disease for American children:

- 1 in 6 children now has a learning disability.[30]
- 1 in 9 suffers from asthma.[31]
- 1 in 10 struggles with a behavioral or mental disorder.[32]
- 1 in 31 is diagnosed with autism.[33]

Is this what progress looks like? In lockstep with the explosion in vaccine recommendations, mandates and compliance rates, American children have become sicker, not healthier.

At every ACIP meeting, the direction is the same: more products, for more people, with fewer options to say no. At the October 2024 meeting, the committee updated both the adult and childhood immunization schedules again, with unanimous votes for nearly all changes. Among the updates: lowering the pneumococcal recommendation from age sixty-five to fifty, adding new meningococcal products to the Vaccines for Children program, and quietly preparing the groundwork for a full pregnancy vaccine schedule. Pregnancy—a natural life process—was even classified as a "medical condition" in the updated schedule.

Notably absent from the conversations? Public health benefit, individualized risk analysis, or long-term outcome data. Instead, the focus was on *uptake*. When childhood recommendations didn't sufficiently target adults at risk for pneumococcal disease, ACIP didn't launch a campaign to reach those adults. They lowered the recommendation age universally. Why? Because blanket recommendations catch the target group and then some—and that "some" represents expanded market share. In this model, every person is a potential end point for pharmaceutical distribution.

So how does the system maintain public trust in this increasingly aggressive vaccine push? It doubles down on fear. And no example better illustrates this than measles.

The Measles Example: A Case Study in Fear, Fiction, and Fallout

When it comes to vaccines, few diseases have been more politicized, weaponized, and misunderstood than measles. If you feel like you hear about measles more than any other illness, despite the sixteen additional diseases included on the childhood immunization schedule, you're not wrong. Measles has been chosen—quite strategically—as the poster child for the global vaccine agenda. According to the World Health Organization, measles cases are the "canary in the coal mine"—a metric used to determine whether global vaccine coverage is slipping.[34] Where there are measles outbreaks, global health authorities see vaccine hesitancy. Measles has become the litmus test for compliance, and as a result, its image has been carefully crafted into a symbol of fear.

At the time of writing this chapter, headlines across the country are shouting about a measles outbreak in Texas that has spread to nearby states like Oklahoma and New Mexico. Just like in the 2015 and 2018 outbreaks, the media has activated the panic script: blame the unvaccinated, warn the public of deadly disease resurgence, and pressure lawmakers and parents to increase vaccine uptake immediately. This time they are even reducing the age that a child is eligible to receive MMR from twelve months to six months.

One particular story, the tragic death of a six-year-old Texas girl, has been used to stoke public fear.[35] The child was unvaccinated and died shortly after being admitted to the hospital while recovering from measles. What few news outlets are reporting, however, is that this child was at the tail end of her illness and had been experiencing difficulty breathing when she was hospitalized. Upon review of the medical records, critical care physician Dr. Pierre Kory concluded that the child did not die of measles itself, but due to medical error and neglecting to administer necessary respiratory treatments—something far more common in US hospitals than the public is ever told.[36]

The truth about measles is more complex than the headlines suggest. For one, measles is a cyclical illness. Historical data from well before the vaccine was introduced in 1963 shows that measles cases rose and fell predictably every two to four years.[37] The idea that measles could be eradicated from Earth with a single vaccine is, according to New York pediatrician Dr. Lawrence Palevsky, a dangerous myth. "The idea that you can eradicate the existence of a measles virus with a vaccine is false," says Palevsky. "It's a lie. It's a myth. And it is propaganda."[38] Despite decades of vaccination, the virus is still here. The biological reality is that viruses mutate, reservoirs persist, and immune responses vary. The belief that the vaccine equals elimination is not grounded in science—it's grounded in ideology.

Even the foundational premise used to justify widespread vaccination— herd immunity—falls apart under scrutiny when applied to measles. The original concept of herd immunity was based on natural exposure: when a high enough percentage of people contract and recover from a viral illness like measles, the illness temporarily runs out of hosts. Natural immunity is robust and lifelong, meaning a recovered individual is unlikely to become reinfected or transmit the virus.

Public health officials have grafted the concept of natural herd immunity onto vaccination, assuming that if enough children receive the measles shot, the community will be protected. But this theory is not supported by the data and is quite frankly mathematically impossible. Studies show that up to 10 percent of children experience primary vaccine failure—they receive the shot but never mount an immune response at all.[39] Others may show an antibody response initially, only to lose measurable "immunity" within six to twelve months. This is why booster shots were introduced. Yet immunity induced by vaccination is not the same as natural immunity; antibodies alone are not proof of long-term protection, and in many cases, they're a poor proxy for true immune resilience.

So why are we seeing fewer acute measles cases today? Some researchers believe it has less to do with eradication and more to do with reclassification. In other words, the *presence of a measles virus illness* cannot be measured solely on one specific *presentation* of the measles virus illness. Many children may no longer present with textbook measles symptoms, but that doesn't mean the virus is gone. There is evidence—found in the autopsies of children who were injured or passed away following MMR vaccination—that the measles virus can linger in the body and even be found in brain tissue.[40] What if we have not eradicated measles but instead converted it into a chronic, low-grade viral burden that our children now carry silently? This issue raises critical questions about the long-term impact of injecting live attenuated viruses into developing immune systems.

Worse still, we have failed to consider the cost of avoiding acute illness. In our zeal to eliminate diseases like measles, we have neglected the growing body of research—and thousands of years of ancestral wisdom— that views acute childhood illness as a natural and even beneficial part of development. Palevsky points to documented developmental leaps that often follow febrile illnesses like measles, mumps, and chickenpox. In Chinese medicine, such illnesses are understood as a way the body purges inherited or maternal acquired toxins. "When a parent in my practice sees their child resolve an acute illness," Palevsky says, "they see the child sleep better, talk better, walk better and behave differently." Medicine has largely lost this appreciation for the healing arc of acute illness, choosing instead to suppress symptoms at all costs. This suppression—often with fever-reducing drugs and antibiotics—may be driving the very epidemic of chronic illness we now see in children.

Consider this: in 1970, autism was estimated to affect 1 in 10,000 children. By 2000, it was 1 in 150. In 2010, 1 in 88. By 2021, it had dropped to 1 in 36. And in some areas today, it's 1 in 12 boys.[41] That is only a single diagnosis of autism. One in 9 children now has ADHD. One in 20 under age five experiences seizures. These are not mild developmental hiccups.

They are signals of widespread immune and neurological dysfunction. We must ask: have we traded short-lived, self-resolving infections like measles for lifelong suffering?

Finally, what is rarely discussed is that measles infection itself—when allowed to run its natural course in healthy children—has been associated with long-term health benefits. Research suggests that childhood febrile illnesses like measles may reduce the incidence of more serious adult diseases such as Hodgkin's lymphoma, cardiac disease, and other certain cancers.[42] And in the broader context of immune education, acute infections help "train" the immune system, prune the nervous system, and allow the body to detoxify. When that process is interfered with or bypassed, especially repeatedly and early in life, we may be disrupting something sacred— and vital—for long-term health. Philosophically when we manipulate the body's innate and intelligent responses, we will have downstream effects. I feel confident in saying that trading childhood illness for long-term dysfunction comes at a great cost. The war on illness has cost entire generations magnitudes of resilience. The law of nature stays true: you cannot suppress biology without consequence.

In short, the measles narrative illustrates the shaky ground within the vaccine program and allows parents to reassess how they choose to approach their child's welfare, development, and overall health.

Vaccine Effectiveness: A Closer Look

We are told vaccines work, but outbreaks still happen in fully vaccinated populations. Mumps outbreaks on naval ships with 100 percent vaccine coverage. Measles in vaccinated school populations. Why? Vaccine failure is real—both primary (the vaccine never worked) and secondary (waning immunity after months or years) failure are a part of the real-world equation. That's why we now need *boosters* for so many vaccines. Look at the polio doses for American children: two months, four months, six months and four years. Artificial immunity, unlike natural immunity, is often short-lived and incomplete.

Polio is another example of both vaccine failure and vaccine-induced disease. Despite the narrative of eradication, most cases of polio globally today are vaccine-derived. In 2022, a man in New York was diagnosed with paralytic polio. The CDC confirmed the infection was caused by a circulating vaccine-derived poliovirus (cVDPV2), not wild-type virus. Wastewater surveillance revealed a wider presence of the same strain—originating from oral polio vaccine shedding.

The oral polio vaccine (OPV), originally developed by Albert Sabin, is still widely used globally due to its low cost and ease of administration. But its live virus component can revert to virulence in the gut and be shed into the environment, spreading vaccine-strain polio. Despite this, global health authorities are developing *new vaccines* to combat the problem created by the first vaccines—a cycle that keeps repeating.

We must ask: Do vaccines build the immune system—or bypass it? If lifelong immunity matters most, why are we relying on short-term antibody responses that fade within years?

The failure of vaccine-induced herd immunity hasn't slowed the expansion of the program—it's accelerated it. When effectiveness is questioned, the solution is not to reassess but to recommend more shots. At the same 2024 ACIP meeting, members floated the idea of reducing the HPV vaccine start age to nine, even while exploring whether one dose might be sufficient instead of two. Multiple new pneumococcal and meningococcal shots are in development for release in 2025, despite confusion even among experts about which version to use and when. The response to public confusion isn't transparency—it's "harmonization" of the language. This means adjusting the phrasing on all schedules to match, so the illusion of clarity remains intact even when the science is murky.

Vaccine Injury and Autism

One of the most controversial and heavily censored conversations is the link between vaccines and autism. The government says the science is settled—but the science has not even been done. Aluminum adjuvants have never been properly studied for their effect on developing brains, yet are found in some of the highest concentrations ever recorded in postmortem studies of brain tissue from individuals with autism.[43]

Among those who are compensated in the vaccine injury court, brain injury is the most common verdict.[44] Autism, although not listed as a "tabled injury," often presents as regressive brain damage—exactly the type of injury compensated for. And if the leading government witness in the Omnibus Autism Proceeding[45] (Dr. Andrew Zimmerman) later admitted that vaccines *can* cause autism in susceptible individuals—and was fired for saying so—why has mainstream media ignored this story? This could be an entire book and there is much information out there on this topic to explore and understand as it relates to metabolic damage, mitochondrial damage, gut damage, neurological damage, and the onset and prevalence of them all.

The Myth of Herd Immunity

We're guilted into vaccinating with the promise of protecting others. But herd immunity was a theory based on natural infection, not artificial vaccination. With 10 percent primary failure and waning immunity, herd immunity is unachievable through vaccines alone.[46] Add to that viral mutation and vaccine strain shedding from the vaccinated, and the premise crumbles further.[47] If herd immunity were real, we wouldn't need boosters. The theory might have worked in nature. Pharma turned it into marketing.

In fact, the immunocompromised are often more vulnerable to vaccinated individuals who are shedding live virus than to the unvaccinated that might be naturally mediating an infection on a cellular level.[48]

The CDC Schedule as Policy—Not Science

The CDC schedule is not law, yet it holds the power of law in nearly every state. Once a vaccine is added, it becomes the basis for school mandates, employer policies, insurance reimbursement, and pharmacist administration rights. As of 2023, rolling updates were added to an annual addendum, and a new "Schedule by Medical Indication" was introduced for children—listing vaccine recommendations for those with chronic conditions like HIV, kidney failure, and even pregnancy.

Once added, vaccines almost never come off. Only two products have ever been removed—DTP and RotaShield—both of which were replaced with similar products.[49] Even those removals took decades and happened under immense public pressure. The HPV vaccine trials, for example, used aluminum-laden adjuvants or old vaccines as the control, not saline placebos, just as DTP was used as the "placebo" when newer versions of the pertussis vaccine were tested.[50] The illusion of scientific rigor collapses when examined closely.

ACIP was founded in 1964 to centralize expert guidance, but the decision-making process is often riddled with conflicts of interest and policy goals that prioritize uptake over individualized care. In 2021, CDC Director Rochelle Walensky overruled ACIP's vote against recommending another COVID booster for healthcare workers—not based on data, but based on political pressure.[51] As she put it: "Even with uncertainty, we must take actions that we anticipate will do the greatest good." When anticipation replaces evidence, we no longer have science-based policy— we have agenda-based medicine.

Parents Are Best Suited to Care for Their Children

Vaccines are not the root issue—the program at large is a symptom of a system that's decided parents can't be trusted to care for their children's immune systems without government mandates. But we say differently. Reclaiming your child's health starts with reclaiming your role as the primary decision-maker and primary health advocate for yourself and your child.

- Understand how the immune system is built and functions brilliantly.
- Learn why each vaccine came to market and how the universal recommendation was justified.
- Know the difference between artificial and natural immunity
- Trust your parental instincts—and the wisdom of the body— when deciding whether to participate in the vaccine program at large and in individual interventions.

In 2024, the chronic disease epidemic finally broke into the national conversation when media figures like Tucker Carlson and candidates like Robert F. Kennedy Jr. and Donald Trump started talking about it openly. Kennedy suspended his campaign to back Trump, citing shared goals of confronting America's chronic illness crisis—a crisis that, for decades, mainstream media refused to acknowledge. The door has now opened to ask: What if the problem isn't lack of access to medicine, but too much forced intervention? What if decades of vaccinating "just to be safe" actually compromised our children's long-term immune health?

Health doesn't come from fear or blind compliance. It comes from empowerment, clarity, and supporting the body's God-given ability to heal, to defend itself, and to build resilience with each "exposure."

The vaccine program has become the foundation of pediatric primary care starting in utero and at Day 1 of life. There is another program that is being built to compete with that foundation: whole genome sequencing of infants. The next chapter is all about genes because it is imperative to understand what is true about your own health and the health of your children. Otherwise, you might be tricked into interventions that treat the existence of a gene as "the root cause" and in turn end up with a cascade of unintended effects and unnecessary suffering.

Once a vaccine is added to the CDC's childhood schedule:

- The federal government purchases and distributes it through the Vaccines for Children (VFC) program
- It becomes exempt from product liability lawsuits under the 1986 Act
- It can be mandated by states for school and daycare attendance
- It becomes a de facto requirement for insurance coverage and employer policies

It's not just medicine. It's an unaccountable, government-backed business model worth hundreds of billions of dollars annually. The public is told it's about public health. The truth is: it's about guaranteed market access—without market consequences.

For readers who wish to explore the full context behind each vaccine on the CDC's childhood shot schedule—including its history, ingredients, development, and the policy framework surrounding it—see *The Vaccine Decision: Every Shot Has a Story* by Valerie Borek, JD, and Leah Wilson, JD. It is an essential companion for parents seeking comprehensive, evidence-based information to make confident and informed decisions.

CHAPTER 5

You Aren't Defective

The "secret of life" is not in our genes, but in the mechanisms that control gene expression.
—Bruce Lipton, cell biologist, pioneer in epigenetics, and researcher at Stanford University School of Medicine

The Lie of Genetic Determinism

We've been told for years that our health is written in our DNA. The story is that if heart disease runs in your family, you're next. If cancer claimed your mother, you're on borrowed time. If you have the "obesity gene," better get used to weight struggles. Then there is one of the most devastating "genetic life sentences" on the rise, if you can even rank them: if your family member had Alzheimer's, your final decades here on Earth won't belong to you. This is genetic determinism. The narrative is powerful, but it is premised upon the shakiest body of science there is and challenged by a large and growing body of scientific research called epigenetics.

If genes truly dictated disease, then we should be seeing the same rates of chronic illness today as we did centuries ago. But that's not the case. Our ancestors didn't suffer from an epidemic of diabetes, autoimmune disorders, neurological disorders, or Alzheimer's.[1] If genetics was a primary driver of disease, these conditions should have been just as prevalent in the human race in the past. Yet today, chronic illness is everywhere. It is hard to justify this rise, over a single lifetime, by pointing to genetic predispositions. It is notable, however, that there have been seismic shifts in our food supply, our stress levels, our exposure to toxins, and our modern way of life. We've been trained to blame our bodies for "its failures" and, as a result, disassociate with our physical being since it is seen as the enemy. You are not broken. You are not defective. You are not trapped by your genes.

The GWAS Disappointment: When the Genetic Dream Collapsed

The genetic revolution was supposed to be the key to unlocking disease. Billions were poured into genome-wide association studies (GWAS), scanning millions of DNA sequences, searching for the elusive "disease genes."[2] The purpose of the inquiry was to decode all future health problems by showing that your genetic code would predict your fate: heart disease, diabetes, cancer, even depression. The reality? A colossal letdown for those who expected DNA alone to decode disease.

When the results rolled in, even the most optimistic researchers had to admit the truth: genes don't control nearly as much as we thought. GWAS studies found that for most diseases, individual genetic variations explained only a tiny fraction of the risk, usually less than 10 percent.[3] Even polygenic risk scores, which combine multiple genetic risk factors, failed to account for much of the variance in chronic disease.[4]

Then Why Do Diseases "Run in Families"?

The argument for "genetic fatalism" or "genetic determinism" often comes from the observation that certain diseases appear to be passed down through generations. This is in fact the experience of many people. It might even be yours, but is it really genetics, or is it the environment and beliefs we inherit? A family that eats the same processed foods, lives under the same stress, and is exposed to the same environmental toxins will often develop the same diseases. But that doesn't mean their genes caused it.[5] It means they unknowingly reinforced the same biological conditions.

A 2014 study in *Nature Genetics* found that 70 to 80 percent of disease risk comes from lifestyle and environment, not inherited genes.[6] Think of genes like a script for a play: the script offers possibilities, but the actors, the director, and the stage setting determine how the story unfolds. Your genetic code is not a verdict. It's a set of instructions waiting for direction.

The Twin Studies That Destroy Genetic Fatalism

There are numerous twin studies that have been conducted to examine the role of genes in various traits, diseases, and behaviors. Twin studies are a fundamental method in genetics research because they help disentangle the effects of genetics (nature) and environment (nurture).

Identical twins share 100 percent of their DNA, yet they often develop completely different diseases.[7] If genes dictated health, twins should be carbon copies of one another in sickness and longevity. But research proves otherwise.

The Danish Twin Registry is one of the oldest and most comprehensive twin databases in the world, established in 1954. It includes twins born in Denmark since 1870, making it a valuable resource for studying aging, longevity, and the genetic basis of various diseases. The registry consists of more than 86,000 twin pairs and has been instrumental in researching the heritability of diseases such as cancer, diabetes, cardiovascular conditions, and psychiatric disorders.[8]

One of the most influential findings from the Danish Twin Registry is its work on longevity and aging. A seminal study in the 1990s analyzed more than 2,800 twin pairs to determine whether genetics or environment played a more significant role in lifespan. The results showed that environmental factors, including lifestyle and diet, played a more significant role than genetics.[9] This means that while genes contribute to longevity, personal health choices and environmental exposures are crucial determinants of lifespan.

Additionally, studies using the registry have provided insights into diseases like Alzheimer's, demonstrating that while genetic predisposition plays a role, environmental triggers and lifestyle factors significantly influence disease onset.[10] This means that a predisposition can exist without ever being triggered.

The Netherlands Twin Register (NTR) was established in 1987 and has grown into one of the largest longitudinal twin studies in the world, tracking more than 200,000 twins and their family members.[11] The study primarily focuses on the heritability of mental health disorders, intelligence, personality traits, and lifestyle behaviors such as physical activity and substance use. Unlike many other twin studies, the NTR also incorporates genome-wide association studies (GWAS) to link genetic variations to behavioral and psychological traits.

NTR has contributed to research on lifestyle choices and health behaviors. It has shown that behaviors such as physical activity, alcohol consumption, and smoking have a genetic component, but they are also significantly influenced by social and cultural environments. For example, twin studies from the NTR suggest that genetic factors explain about 50 percent of the variation in physical activity levels, indicating that while some people may be naturally inclined to be more active, external influences like upbringing and education also play a critical role.[12]

The Netherlands Twin Register continues to be at the forefront of behavioral genetics research, helping to refine our understanding of how genes and environment interact in shaping human health, cognition, and behavior. With ongoing studies incorporating advanced genetic sequencing and neuroimaging, the NTR is poised to provide even more groundbreaking insights into the complexities of human development.

The Swedish twin registry was used to look at twins separated at birth and reared apart. Some twins developed the same conditions, but many had radically different health outcomes, including in instances like cardiovascular disease and obesity that are thought to be highly genetic.[13]

Their genes were the same, but their environments, stress levels, and habits were different. Genes are merely potential. How you live is ultimately the deciding factor.

Epigenetics and the Ghosts of Starvation

There are two different bodies of science when it comes to genetics: mainstream genetics used by Medicine and epigenetics. You cannot reconcile sciences that look through different lenses: one casts genes as fate, the other treats them as responsive to environment, thought, and behavior. Epigenetics is a different paradigm for how life is influenced and expressed. This distinction isn't just theoretical; it has played out in history in stark, measurable ways. If genes were destiny, the children born during the Dutch Hunger Winter of 1944 should have followed a predictable genetic script. They did not. What happened instead revealed how much the environment, not genetic code alone, shapes health.

During this Nazi-imposed famine, pregnant women ate very little. Their children might have been expected to be born small and then catch up. Instead, they carried lifelong biological scars. Researchers reported higher rates of obesity, diabetes, cardiovascular disease, and mental health problems decades later in those exposed in utero.[14] Some effects were observed in the next generation without any change to DNA sequence.[15] What changed was which genes were turned on or off, a process studied in the field of epigenetics.

Epigenetics is the biological control system that determines which genes are expressed and which remain silent. Think of your DNA as the keys on a piano; epigenetics is the pianist deciding which notes to play and which to mute. Your genes hold potential, but your environment (your food, stress levels, toxins, movement, and even your thoughts) guides how that potential is expressed. Unlike genetic mutations, which alter the DNA sequence, epigenetic changes are reversible and strongly influenced by lifestyle. In other words, your body is continually rewriting its biological script based on the signals you send it.

In the case of the Dutch Hunger Winter, prenatal famine exposure appears to have reprogrammed metabolism, priming these children to store fat and hold on to calories as if another famine were imminent. This was not about bad genes. It was about how external factors such as stress, toxins, and nutrition determine whether you express vitality or dysfunction. The Dutch Hunger Winter challenged genetic determinism and affirmed a long-standing truth: your health is not simply inherited; it is cultivated.

What about Genetic Mutations?

Studies suggest that many genetic mutations are not merely random errors but, in most cases, adaptive responses to environmental stressors, much like how plants alter gene expression to survive in toxic soil. However, not all mutations are adaptive; some arise from replication errors from external damage. The concept of Penetrance is the chance that a gene change will lead to a specific condition. It shows that most conditions are not inevitable. Huntington's disease is one of the few with nearly 100 percent penetrance, meaning the mutation almost always results in the disease.[16] Even conditions with very high penetrance, like achondroplasia (a genetic form of dwarfism), do not always show up in every person who carries the gene. Yet gene-centered Medicine often treats every genetic change as if it guarantees disease, overlooking how environment, nutrition, and epigenetic factors influence which genes turn on or off. High penetrance is the exception, not the rule. For nearly all chronic diseases (heart disease, diabetes, cancer, obesity, Alzheimer's, autoimmune disorders), genetics may create a predisposition, but they have unknown penetrance. Your environment, habits, and mindset decide whether those genes activate. A 2019 study in *Cell Metabolism* found that people with genetic markers for Type 2 diabetes could completely reverse their risk through diet and lifestyle changes.[17] The genes didn't change. Their expression did. Your DNA is a blueprint. But you are the builder.

The Agouti Mice Experiment: More Proof That Genes Are Not Destiny

One of the most striking examples of epigenetics in action comes from a groundbreaking study on Agouti mice. These mice carry a gene known as Agouti, which, when fully expressed, makes them obese, yellow-furred, and prone to diabetes and cancer. For years, scientists believed this condition was purely genetic; after all, generation after generation of Agouti mice exhibited the same characteristics. But what happened when researchers altered the diet of pregnant Agouti mice?

A study published in *Molecular and Cellular Biology* found that by simply changing the diet of the mother during pregnancy (adding methyl-rich nutrients like folate and B vitamins), her offspring were born lean, brown, and free of disease.[18] The genetic code in these mice never changed. The only thing that changed was which genes were turned on and off based on environmental factors (in this case, nutrition). If a mouse can escape genetic "destiny" through environmental change, imagine what's possible for you.

The Angelina Jolie Effect

Perhaps nowhere is genetic fear more obvious than in the BRCA1/2 gene story. This in large part due to the public visibility of the issue following high-profile cases that brought attention to hereditary cancer risks for women. In 2013, Angelina Jolie disclosed that she tested positive for a BRCA1 mutation and publicized her choice to have a preventative bilateral mastectomy. A 2001 study published in the *New England Journal of Medicine* reported that approximately 50 percent of women with these mutations opted for prophylactic bilateral mastectomy.[19] A study found that preventative mastectomy rates have tripled over the last two decades, with a significant increase following Jolie's announcement.[20] This is a phenomenon termed the "Angelina Jolie effect."

Women who test positive for these genes are often told they have up to an 87 percent chance of developing breast cancer.[21] Preventive mastectomies are encouraged, even when no cancer is present. But how is that 87 percent number calculated? And is it an accurate reflection of a woman's true risk? The answer is complicated, and the statistic is deeply flawed.

The statistic that BRCA1/2 carriers have up to an 87 percent lifetime risk of developing breast cancer comes from a 1990 study published in *Science* by Mary-Claire King, the same researcher who first identified the BRCA1 gene in 1990.[22] The study analyzed a group of women from high-risk families, meaning families that already had multiple members diagnosed with breast or ovarian cancer.

Here's the key problem: the study examined a highly selective group: women with strong family histories of breast cancer. In other words, the participants were already in an environment with a high likelihood of disease. When researchers start with a group that has above-average risk and then analyze their genes, the results can be skewed. The study did not measure all women with BRCA mutations; it looked only at those from families where breast cancer was common.

This would be like studying a group of smokers and concluding they have an 87 percent risk of lung cancer, then assuming that risk applies to all people, including nonsmokers. The selection bias is glaring. When subsequent studies analyzed BRCA carriers from the general population, rather than from high-risk families, the numbers looked very different.

- A 2003 study in the *New England Journal of Medicine* found that BRCA1/2 mutation carriers without a strong family history of breast cancer had a significantly lower risk, around 40 percent, not 87 percent.[23]
- A 2008 study in the *Journal of the National Cancer Institute* further confirmed that environment, lifestyle, and dietary factors dramatically influenced risk among BRCA carriers, showing that women who maintained a healthy weight, exercised regularly, and did not smoke had far lower cancer rates than those who did not.[24]

It doesn't stop with a life-altering preventative surgery. What are the implications for your lymphatic flow, your hormones, your confidence, your sexual relations? There is a cost to these choices, and it is not the only choice. The loudest voice in this space shapes the common understanding that young women should live in fear of the cancers of their mothers and grandmothers. If a woman even mentions the loss of her loved one due to female cancers, you can almost guarantee that unsolicited fear and pity will be foisted upon her by not only doctors but also family, friends, and colleagues.

The BRCA fear narrative is mostly an American construct. In other parts of the world, BRCA carriers have dramatically different cancer risks.

Why the 87 Percent Statistic Persists

Despite clear evidence that the true risk for BRCA carriers varies dramatically based on lifestyle and environment, the 87 percent figure is still widely used. Why? Well, consider that preventive mastectomies, hysterectomies, and aggressive monitoring create a multibillion-dollar industry for hospitals, surgeons, and pharmaceutical companies. Angelina Jolie's 2013 double mastectomy, which she publicized as a preventive measure due to her BRCA status, caused BRCA testing rates to skyrocket by 64 percent in the United States within a few months of her announcement.[25]

This isn't to say that all women who opt for these procedures are in error. But they deserve full, unbiased information, not fear-based statistics.

The Real Risk for BRCA Carriers

If you are a BRCA carrier, your actual risk of developing cancer is highly dependent on your lifestyle, diet, and environment.

Instead of focusing on a blanket 87 percent statistic, a more accurate assessment would be:

- Are you consuming an anti-inflammatory, nutrient-dense diet? (chapters 10 and 19)
- Are you minimizing your exposure to environmental toxins, endocrine disruptors, and xenoestrogens? (chapters 11, 12 and 19)
- Are you chronically stressed, or do you prioritize peace management? (chapters 9 and 16)
- Do you engage in regular physical activity? (chapter 9)

Each of these factors has been shown to significantly impact BRCA gene expression. A 2013 study in *JAMA* found that women with BRCA mutations who exercised, ate well, and avoided smoking had dramatically lower rates of breast cancer than those who didn't.[26]

Turned On. Turned Off.

I often hear people ask, if I've already "turned on" "bad genes" can I reverse it? Absolutely. Just as poor choices can activate disease-promoting genes, the right conditions can silence them. Your body is constantly replacing cells. Every day, millions of new cells are created, and every few years, nearly every cell in your body is replaced. That means you have a constant opportunity to reprogram your biology. A study showed that lifestyle changes, particularly food, stress reduction (peace management), and fasting, can reverse harmful gene expression in as little as three months.[27]

Fear as a Disease Trigger: The Nocebo Effect

One of the biggest challenges with believing you are genetically flawed, mutated, or broken is that those beliefs alone can make you sick. This is the Nocebo Effect, the opposite of the Placebo Effect.

A 2007 study in *The Lancet* found that people who believed they were at high risk for heart disease were four times more likely to die from it, even when their actual health markers were normal.[28] Another study showed that women told they had a genetic risk for obesity gained more weight than those who weren't told, despite following the same diet.[29]

Fear isn't just psychological, it's biochemical. Chronic fear floods the body with stress hormones, weakens the immune system, and alters gene expression.[30] We'll explore this concept further in chapter 8, but for now, ask yourself: Are you carrying a fear of disease that is shaping your health outcomes?

Bruce Lipton's statement, "Your biology is controlled by your thoughts. Your cells are listening to your beliefs," is a powerful encapsulation of the core principle of epigenetics, the idea that our genes are not rigid, deterministic blueprints, but rather dynamic systems influenced by our environment, lifestyle, and, most strikingly, our perceptions and beliefs. Our thoughts and beliefs, especially when deeply ingrained, play a pivotal role in regulating gene expression.

In other words, you can think of your mind as your biological regulator. The brain is not just an organ of cognition; it is a biochemical command center that constantly communicates with the body. Thoughts generate neurochemical signals that influence our hormonal balance, immune function, and stress response, all of which have profound effects on how our genes are activated or silenced.

For example:

- **Chronic stress** activates genes linked to inflammation and disease, increasing susceptibility to conditions like cardiovascular disease and autoimmune disorders.
- **Positive beliefs and gratitude** are shown to enhance the expression of genes associated with immune strength, longevity, and resilience.

It is worth repeating, your genes are a blueprint, but you are the builder. The question is: Are you going to keep following the old blueprint, or are you ready to draft a new one?

The Genetic Trap: Whole Genome Sequencing of Newborns

For decades, newborn screening has been a standard tool used to check for serious but treatable conditions in infants, such as phenylketonuria (PKU), sickle cell disease, cystic fibrosis, hypothyroidism, and MCAD deficiency. Initially, screening was limited to a handful of well-understood diseases. However, advances in AI and whole genome sequencing have dramatically expanded the scope.

Today, states screen for thirty to sixty conditions, and with emerging technologies, the potential exists to screen for over 7,000 genetic diseases at birth using whole genome sequencing (WGS).[31] Enthusiasts of this shift frame it as an exciting leap from limited screening into full-scale genome sequencing, a transformation that is no longer theoretical, it is happening now. But behind the promises of early intervention and precision medicine lie profound ethical, financial, and societal concerns that could redefine the life of the tested children and their families.

One of the most glaring issues is the financial incentive behind mass WGS for newborns. The pharmaceutical industry has recognized this as an unprecedented opportunity, with over five hundred new genetic-based drugs in development.[32] The Orphan Drug Act, originally designed to fast-track treatments for rare diseases, grants market exclusivity to drug makers for seven years. However, when screening expands to test every newborn for thousands of genetic variations, the likelihood of finding something "wrong" increases dramatically. Like a whole-body MRI that reveals benign anomalies, WGS has the potential to medicalize normal variations, leading to unnecessary interventions in your new baby and costly treatments.

Take Krabbe disease as an example, a rare genetic condition characterized by severe neurological deterioration. Symptoms such as irritability, feeding difficulties, and regression from developmental milestones mirror what some would describe as vaccine injury.[33] Yet, once a gene variant is identified, the next step often leads to gene-altering therapies.

What Did We Learn from Jesse Gelsinger's Death in 1999?

Eighteen-year-old Jesse Gelsinger was living a normal life and managing a genetic condition called ornithine transcarbamylase deficiency (OTCD) with medication and a low-protein diet. He entered a safety trial for gene therapy to treat the metabolic disorder. Jesse passed four days after the gene therapy. Jesse and his parents were not told that other participants had experienced severe effects or that animals had died in the animal trials. His death sent shock waves through the research community. Gene therapy research was halted, and some researchers even said the field of gene therapy just went away after his death.[34]

Fast-forward twenty years and we have Zolgensma, a gene therapy for spinal muscular atrophy, on the market priced at $2.1 million per injection. Despite the drug being one of the most expensive in the world, the data supporting its approval was later found to be inaccurate: it initially reported that six out of seven mice survived, when in fact six out of seven died.[35] Despite acknowledging the corrupted data, the FDA allowed the drug to remain on the market for the rare disease; it remains available as of this writing.

Beyond cost and questionable data, the lack of transparency in WGS raises further concerns. Unlike traditional diagnostic tests where doctors interpret the results, genetic sequencing operates through proprietary algorithms owned by a single dominant player in the industry, Illumina, a US-based company with ties to China that holds a near-monopoly on the process.[36] This means that diagnoses and prognoses for newborns are dictated by an algorithm rather than a physician's clinical judgment.

Genetic screening programs are often structured as opt-out rather than opt-in, meaning parents must actively refuse testing, sometimes under pressure from medical authorities. Families who decline screening or treatments may be accused of medical neglect, which can trigger intervention by child protective services. This trend has already appeared in cases involving cancer, ADHD, depression, and, more recently, gender dysphoria.

Science or Worldview?

The deeper danger is not just the screening technology itself, but the worldview it reflects. Genetic determinism is built on a low view of the human body, as if we are born faulty and in need of correction. It is the belief that our biology is permanently flawed and must be managed from the outside in. This perspective fuels a fear-based response to new life, convincing parents that their healthy child is a ticking time bomb. It drives them toward high-cost, high-risk interventions while ignoring the profound impact of nutrients, minerals, the microbiome, and the nervous system, all of which are designed to support life, not fear it.

Real-world examples challenge genetic determinism or the gene theory. For instance, a child diagnosed with a genetic immunodeficiency was told he would never produce antibodies and required $16,000-per-month infusions. Yet, after receiving chiropractic care and nutrient support, his immune system began producing antibodies on its own, an outcome the genetic diagnosis deemed impossible. The mention of chiropractic and gene expression might feel disconnected, but studies show that long-term chiropractic patients exhibit higher levels of serum thiols, a marker of DNA repair, independent of diet or supplements.[37] This is just one of the thousands of examples that highlight the fact that genes do not dictate fate, and the body's capacity for healing is far greater than we've been led to believe.

As newborn WGS grows, are we advancing medicine or creating a profit-driven system that turns human differences into diagnoses? The push toward mass genetic screening is not just a technological shift, it is an ideological one, reinforcing a worldview where life's trajectory is determined at birth and managed through pharmaceuticals. It places faith in man's prognosis over God's design, fostering fear instead of confidence in the body's innate wisdom. If we fail to challenge this framework, we risk allowing an entire generation to be stripped of the vitalism that defines true health.

Genetics Is One of the Primary Foundations of Medicine

The use of genetic testing, and genetic reasons for treatment, has become common in Medicine and even in integrative and holistic care. From prenatal screening to cancer risk assessments, genetics now plays a central role in medical decisions, even though most gene changes do not guarantee disease. Whether a gene actually causes illness (penetrance) varies widely, and when it does, the effects can range from mild to severe.

Genetics is also the driving force for more "personalized medicine." In other words, using your genes to determine what medications you need and how you will respond to those medications. Conditions once considered primarily environmental or lifestyle-driven, such as obesity and mental health disorders, are now being linked to genetic predispositions, shifting the narrative toward medical and pharmaceutical interventions based on genetic markers instead of long-term solutions and accountability for health outcomes. It is a principle of success to believe that our decisions make a difference, not that one is a victim to a given set of fixed circumstances. We may not control every variable, but we are not slaves to our genes. To believe otherwise is to surrender stewardship of the body to a system that profits from our resignation.

The widespread reliance on genetic data for medical decision-making raises critical questions about the balance between prevention and overreach. While genetics plays a role, the environment, lifestyle, and epigenetic factors also have the most significant impact on genetic expression.

The concern is that genetic testing could lead to a deterministic mindset, where individuals are told they are destined for disease rather than empowered with ways to influence their health outcomes. This shift in focus can justify aggressive medical interventions, such as prophylactic surgeries, lifelong medications, or gene-editing technologies, even when alternative, noninvasive approaches might be equally effective. As genetic testing becomes more deeply embedded in medicine, a broader discussion is needed about its limitations, ethical considerations, and the extent to which genetic findings should dictate medical decisions.

But don't wait for Medicine to find its way. History tells us the pattern. The pendulum swings hard in one direction. People suffer. The damage becomes undeniable. Only then does the system slowly correct itself. That process can take decades. While Medicine sorts itself out, you have a choice right now. Genes may load the gun, but they do not pull the trigger. You are not bound to a script. You help write and rewrite it every single day. The question is, what are you writing today?

Rewriting the Blueprint

Most people have never questioned their beliefs about genetics. It's time to challenge the narrative you've been given. If genetic determinism isn't the whole story, then what about the conditions that seem to defy everything we've said so far like cancer and autoimmunity? For many, these diagnoses feel like the body's ultimate betrayal, proof that it has gone rogue. But what if the opposite is true? What if cancer and autoimmunity are not exceptions to the body's design, but expressions of intelligent adaptations to a toxic, stressed environment? In the chapters ahead, we'll step into some of the most feared terrain in all of Medicine, uncover the myths that have shaped our understanding, and reveal a radically different perspective: one that sees even these "worst-case scenarios" not as death sentences, but as invitations to restore the terrain, reclaim hope, and align with the body's remarkable capacity to heal.

CHAPTER 6

Are Cancer and Autoimmunity Exceptions?

Cancer is not a genetic disease. Cancer is a metabolic disease. It's the body's attempt to survive.
—Dr. Thomas N. Seyfried, PhD (professor of biology, Boston College; author of *Cancer as a Metabolic Disease*)

By now, you may be seeing the body in a new light: not as something broken to be fixed, but as something brilliantly designed to heal, adapt, and survive. With that understanding comes a sense of freedom: the freedom to stop suppressing symptoms, stop warring against your body, stop managing disease, and start supporting the body with trust and intention.

But then there's cancer.

This is where many people hit a wall. Cancer has touched too many of us, up close, personal, and painfully. We've watched loved ones endure unbearable suffering, devastating treatments, and outcomes that no one deserves. Even those who live healthy, natural lives and hold a deep faith in and knowledge of the body's wisdom often wrestle with a quiet thought: "Cancer feels like the exception." And that's understandable. But what if it's not the exception? What if we've just inherited the wrong story?

The good news is, you don't have to wait for a diagnosis to change how you care for your body. You can build a foundation now, physically, mentally, and spiritually, that makes you stronger, not more afraid. And if cancer does come, there are better ways to respond than what most people are offered. There are providers, strategies, and frameworks that don't pit you against your own body but work with it. This chapter will challenge what you believe about cancer. And for most people, that belief needs to be challenged.

If we want to break the cycle of suffering in our families, we have to question the assumptions we've inherited. Beliefs aren't formed in a vacuum. They are shaped by media headlines, pharmaceutical marketing, government campaigns, and well-meaning doctors. But most of all, they are shaped by experience, especially when that experience is cancer. And the story we believed going in often determines how we interpret what happened next.

That's why we can't afford to stay passive. You don't need to become a cancer researcher, but you do need to understand the basics. Because the moment you realize that cancer and autoimmunity might not be random acts of destruction but intelligent responses to a deeper imbalance is the moment everything begins to shift.

The Attack on Self?

As it stands today, cancer remains the ultimate diagnosis of fear. It looms larger than life. Unfortunately, the longer you live and the more people you love, the more likely you are to encounter it. I've been in rooms where people still whisper about it, calling it "the big C," too afraid to even say the word aloud. That's how deep the fear runs.

The narrative is well-worn: your body has gone rogue, mutated beyond control, and is now at war with itself. It's a terrifying story. But what if it's the wrong one? What if cancer isn't an exception to the body's intelligence, but an expression of it?

That shift alone changes everything. It's the same with autoimmunity. We've been told for decades that autoimmune conditions are the body "attacking itself," a biological betrayal. But that theory is outdated and damaging. It leads to treatments that suppress the immune system, rather than asking: what is the body actually trying to do?

You can see where this is going. Your understanding shapes your response. And your response determines whether you pursue healing or settle for managing a label. Cancer and autoimmunity aren't random acts of destruction. They are intelligent survival responses: the body adapting to a toxic, depleted, and stressed environment in an effort to sustain itself, even when conditions are not conducive to life.

To pursue true healing, we have to see the body rightly. We have to understand health, not just disease. And we must begin to honor this truth: Your body, your mind, and your spirit are not separate. How you care for your body is inseparable from how you live, and how you live is inseparable from what you believe. But what if the beliefs you hold were shaped by more than just personal experience? What if the entire cancer narrative was forged through politics, profit, and a war that never should have been waged?

The War on Cancer: Fifty-Plus Years of Losing

In 1971, President Nixon declared war on cancer. It was framed as a moon-shot moment: "the same way we put a man on the moon, we are going to eradicate cancer."[1] The government poured billions into research, and trillions have been spent since. But what have we gained? We're still losing.

Incidence of cancer increased sharply through the 1980s and 1990s according to Surveillance, Epidemiology, and End Results data from the National Cancer Institute.[2] Overall cancer incidence rose from about 1 in 250 in the 1970s to 1 in 200 by the 1990s. Childhood cancer rates also increased steadily and became more common among children starting in the 1970s and 1980s. That's a staggering 25 percent increase in two decades following Nixon's declaration. The latest SEER/NCI data shows 1 in 2 men will be diagnosed with cancer in their lifetime and 1 in 3 women.[3] Cancer is now the second leading cause of death worldwide, despite the "advancements" in chemotherapy, radiation, and immunotherapy. The death toll keeps rising, the treatments remain brutal, and we're left asking: why hasn't all this money solved the problem? We have been fighting the wrong battle: fighting against the body instead of honoring its warnings and fighting for healing.

Several factors after 1970 may have contributed to the surge. DDT was widely used into the early 1970s,[4] and other persistent pollutants, including PCBs and dioxins, continued to accumulate in people and the environment.[5] The vaccine schedule expanded dramatically after 1986, and there have been concerns about links to cancer development.[6] No long-term carcinogenicity studies have been done on the vaccine schedule or on most individual vaccines. In addition, the rise in overmedicalization disrupting microbiomes and immune function started in the 1970s.[7]

And in the 1980s there was a surge in added sugar and ultra-processed foods in the American diet.[8] Stack all of that on top of Rockefeller Medicine, where symptoms were silenced, the body was drugged into submission, and natural healing was dismissed as quackery,[9] and you get the perfect storm. We are not just losing a war. We are standing in the wreckage of a war fought on the wrong battlefield.

A War Built on the Wrong Foundation

Cancer care evolved within the same allopathic system that Rockefeller-era Medicine put in place. That system was never designed to cure. It was designed to pharmaceuticalize disease, control medical education, and turn patients into lifelong customers.

By the time Nixon's War on Cancer was declared, Rockefeller Medicine was already in full control. The Flexner Report of 1910 had wiped out natural medicine and reshaped medical schools to focus solely on pharmaceuticals and surgery. Any approach to cancer that didn't fit this model was erased.

The National Cancer Act of 1971 was not about curing cancer; it was about centralizing control over cancer research and treatment. Instead of looking at cancer as a metabolic disease, a toxicity issue, or a symptom of a failing terrain, it was framed as a genetic malfunction, something we had to fight, kill, and destroy.

And who shaped that narrative?

- The American Cancer Society, an organization with deep ties to the pharmaceutical industry.
- The National Cancer Institute, which funds research that overwhelmingly supports drug-based treatments.
- Big Pharma and the American Medical Association, the policy and political arm of modern Medicine, ensured that only

"approved" cancer treatments, such as chemotherapy, radiation, and surgery, would be recognized as legitimate.

From that moment on, the conversation was controlled. No alternative viewpoints allowed.

The People Who Fell through the Cracks

But here's the thing: not everyone bought into this system.

For decades, people have sought cancer care outside the allopathic model, not because they are desperate or reckless but because they have watched loved ones suffer through chemo and radiation, only to see the cancer return even stronger. Others have worked in the medical system and seen firsthand how little success conventional treatments often achieve. Then there are those who have been harmed by the cancer system itself, left sicker, weaker, and with no answers except "Let's try another round." And, of course, there are those who simply do not think the mainstream options make sense.

These are the people who turn to integrative clinics, metabolic therapies, and alternative cancer treatments, the very approaches that were written out of the medical system over a century ago. And what does the mainstream do? It mocks them. It calls them quacks. It threatens their licenses. It shuts them down.

Yet, if the war was so successful, why are people running from the system in droves, searching for "alternative" answers?

The Same Failed Playbook for Fifty Years

Modern oncology still treats cancer as the enemy, something to cut out, poison, or burn away. That's why the three main treatments haven't changed much in decades:

1. Surgery—**Cut** the tumor out.
2. Chemotherapy—**Poison** the cancer cells (and healthy ones too).
3. Radiation—**Burn** the tumor and potentially the surrounding areas into oblivion.

These treatments focus entirely on treating cancer, never addressing *why it developed in the first place*. And because of that, recurrence rates remain high, survival rates barely budge, and cancer continues to rise. If the standard treatments were truly solving the problem, wouldn't we be seeing a decline in cancer instead of an explosion?

Cancer Surgery: Cutting the Tumor, but at What Cost?

When most people hear "cancer treatment," they think of surgery. Cut it out, get rid of it, problem solved, right? You often hear, "we were able to get it all." That's the prevailing belief. The tumor is seen as the enemy, and surgery is the weapon used to take it down. But what if cutting out the tumor doesn't actually solve the problem? What if, in some cases, it makes things worse?

Cancer surgery does one thing well: it reduces what's called the *tumor load*, or the amount of cancerous tissue present in the body. In certain situations, this can be helpful or necessary. For example, if a large tumor is physically compressing a vital organ, blocking blood flow, or interfering with normal body function, removing it may provide immediate relief and give the body a better chance to begin the healing process.

However, emerging research is raising concern about an unintended consequence of surgery: the potential to increase the risk of *metastasis*.[10] Metastasis occurs when cancer cells leave the original tumor and travel to the bones, brain, lungs, liver, or other organs, where they form new tumors.[11] This process makes the disease far more difficult to treat and is the main reason cancer becomes life-threatening.

How Surgery May Increase Cancer Spread

Surgery is often framed as a "cure," but the reality is more complicated. Research shows that tumor removal can actually increase the likelihood of cancer spreading to other areas of the body.[12] Here's why:

- When a tumor is surgically removed, millions of cancer cells can be released into the bloodstream. These free-floating cells are looking for a new place to latch on to, and surgery may actually make it easier for them to stick to other tissues.[13]

- Surgery is a massive stressor on the body. Postsurgical immune suppression is well-documented, and it can last for weeks. If the immune system was already struggling to keep cancer cells in check, this window of suppression gives remaining cancer cells the chance to grow unchecked.[14]
- Angiogenesis, the growth of new blood vessels, supports wound repair. In cancer, it also fuels tumor growth by increasing blood flow to cancer cells. Surgery can set off healing responses that stimulate angiogenesis in residual cancer cells.[15]
- Surgery is trauma, and trauma sparks an inflammatory response. Cancer thrives in an inflamed environment. The stress response, tissue damage, and cytokine release following surgery may accelerate the conditions that allowed cancer to grow in the first place.[16]

There is a reason the cells go into an adaptive state and tumors form. So cutting out the tumor and never addressing why it was there in the first place makes no sense, yet the industry maintains this practice still today. It is devastating to hear from the woman who got a double mastectomy to fight cancer, and three years later the tumors are back, only now under her armpits.[17]

The Myth of Spare Body Parts

Cancer surgery is just one expression of a deeper, misguided philosophy in Medicine: *when the body part becomes a problem, cut it out. You didn't need it anyway.*

This belief, that healing comes through removal, has driven everything from breast and thyroid removals to prophylactic organ extractions such as Angelina Jolie's widely publicized mastectomy and oophorectomy. These procedures are praised as brave and preventive, yet they follow a fear-based script written by genetic determinism. This thinking is not just flawed; it is barbaric.

Take tonsillectomies and adenoidectomies. For decades, these surgeries have been performed on children as a "routine" fix for common infections. But tonsils and adenoids are not mistakes of nature. They are lymphatic tissues, vital parts of the body's immune defense, placed at the critical intersection of the respiratory and digestive systems. To cut them out without understanding their function is like removing your home's smoke detectors because they keep going off.

A groundbreaking 2018 study of 1.2 million Danish children found that those who had their tonsils or adenoids removed before age nine had dramatically higher long-term risks of developing respiratory diseases, allergies, infections, and immune dysfunction.[18] In other words, the very procedures meant to prevent illness ended up making people sicker. These surgeries didn't solve the underlying issue. They suppressed a symptom by sacrificing the body's own defenses.

Sayer Ji, founder of GreenMedInfo, put it bluntly: "The conventional model of medicine still treats organs as replaceable parts in a malfunctioning machine. But the body isn't a machine—it's a living ecosystem. And no part is expendable."[19] His story of lifelong health struggles after childhood adenoid removal only underscores the real cost of this cut-first, ask-questions-later approach.

Whether it's tonsils, breasts, prostates, or thyroids, we must ask: What kind of medicine amputates the immune system in order to save it? What kind of science ignores the intelligence of the body to force a symptom into silence?

Removing a symptom does not equal healing. In fact, it may set the body further back. We're not designed with spare parts. Every organ plays a role in the symphony of health, and we must stop silencing the instruments just because the music sounds off.

If we want to truly heal, we must ask better questions. Instead of, "What can we cut out?" The question must be: "What is the body trying to do, and how can we support it?" There can be far worse hardships down the road if we don't get to the root cause of what the body is telling us and simply move on after cutting out the problem.

Chemotherapy: The Reality

Some cancers respond well to chemotherapy. Testicular cancer and Hodgkin's lymphoma are two examples. In these cases, the treatment can significantly improve survival rates.[20] But for most cancers, the numbers tell a different story.

While Medicine touts the benefits of chemotherapy as a cornerstone of cancer treatment, the overall impact on survival is modest at best. A 2004 study published in *Clinical Oncology* analyzed twenty-two major adult malignancies and found that chemotherapy contributed only 2.1 percent to five-year survival rates in the United States and 2.3 percent in Australia.[21] And yet, this remains the number one form of treatment in conventional oncology.

But where did chemotherapy even come from? Its origins aren't exactly inspiring.

Chemotherapy didn't start in a lab dedicated to healing, it started on the battlefield. During World War I, mustard gas was used as a chemical weapon, causing horrific burns and lung damage.[22] Decades later, during World War II, researchers studying its effects on soldiers noticed something interesting: mustard gas severely suppressed white blood cell production.[23] This led scientists at Yale in the 1940s to explore its potential as a treatment for blood cancers like lymphoma and leukemia, where uncontrolled white blood cell growth was the problem.[24]

The first official chemotherapy drug, mustine (mechlorethamine), was literally derived from mustard gas.[25] It worked by damaging DNA and stopping cells from dividing, a mechanism that became the basis for most chemotherapy drugs that followed.[26] The logic was simple: because cancer cells divide rapidly, a drug that targets dividing cells should kill them. In reality, it also kills healthy cells and disrupts the microbiome, causing dysbiosis (unhealthy shift in gut bacteria).

Chemotherapy is often compared to dropping a nuclear bomb on the body. It doesn't just target cancer cells; it also destroys healthy, fast-dividing cells, including those in the gut, immune system, and hair follicles. That's why nausea, extreme fatigue, immune suppression, and hair loss are so common with treatment.

Yes, chemotherapy can shrink tumors. But at what cost? If survival rates across most cancers hover around 2.1 percent improvement, is it worth the devastation it brings to the rest of the body?[27]

With numbers that low, the real question isn't "How do we improve chemotherapy?" but rather, "Why is this still the standard approach?"

Radiation: Killing Cancer, but at What Cost?

Radiation therapy is designed with one goal in mind: destroy cancer cells by blasting them with high-energy radiation. It does this by damaging the DNA inside cancer cells, making it impossible for them to divide and grow.[28] The intent is clear: target the tumor, shrink it, and stop its spread. In some cases, it does exactly that.

Just like chemotherapy, radiation does not only target cancer cells. It damages everything in its path, including healthy tissues, immune cells, and the systems that protect you. If you have seen someone go through radiation, you have seen the side effects: burned skin, extreme fatigue, weakened immunity, and long-term tissue damage. Yes, radiation can reduce tumor burden, but at what cost to the body's ability to heal? In some cases, new tumors are later found near the area that was irradiated.[29]

The mainstream cancer model assumes that destroying the tumor is the same as solving the problem. Cancer is not just a mass of rogue cells; it is an adaptive response to an unhealthy environment. Here's why radiation might not be the clean-cut solution it's sold as:

- Your immune system is the primary defense against cancer, constantly identifying and eliminating rogue cells. Radiation damages the immune system by killing white blood cells and weakening bone marrow function, leaving the door wide open for cancer to return.[30]
- Radiation doesn't only hit the tumor. The healthy tissue surrounding it takes a massive hit, leading to scar tissue, chronic inflammation, and long-term damage to vital organs.[31]
- Cancer cells are incredibly adaptive. When exposed to a stressful, toxic environment (like radiation), they can mutate, becoming more aggressive and resistant to treatment.[32] This is why some people undergo radiation, see initial improvement, and then get hit with a more malignant cancer later.
- Research suggests that radiation can actually induce genetic mutations in surrounding cells, increasing the risk of secondary cancers down the line.[33] In other words, the treatment itself may create the very disease it's trying to eliminate.

Let's put it this way: radiation is like throwing a grenade into a room full of rats. Yes, the rats (cancer cells) may die. But what's left of the room? The walls are scorched, the foundation is cracked, and if you don't rebuild it, what happens? More destruction. More opportunity for disease to take root again.

This is where conventional oncology goes wrong: it focuses on killing cancer, not on restoring health.

Kill the Cancer, or Restore the Body?

And while these treatments sometimes shrink tumors, they don't address the real issue: what caused cancer in the first place? What was my body trying to adapt to? What needed to change for it to no longer be in survival mode?

That's why recurrence rates remain so high. We call it remission, but in reality, we've often just suppressed the symptom without resolving the cause. The body was silenced, but nothing meaningful changed. And if the person walks away believing it was all just bad luck or bad genes, they're left with no road map and no responsibility, only fear.

Meanwhile, cancer rates have skyrocketed since industrialization. According to the American Cancer Society, as of 2022, an American has a 1 in 3 chance of developing cancer in their lifetime and a 1 in 6 chance of dying from cancer.[34] What changed? Our environment. Our food. Our toxic load. We've created a world that promotes cancer.

If You Choose Conventional Treatments, You Have to Rebuild

If you choose conventional, you have to go into repair mode immediately. That means you must rebuild the immune system, heal the damaged tissue, and detoxify the system. This certainly won't mitigate all the damage that was done but it will certainly help. Regardless, in order to prevent or beat something, you have to first know what it is. And cancer is not exactly what you've been told.

A transformative story that beautifully illustrates the power of addressing root causes in healing is Liana Werner-Gray, the bestselling author of *Cancer Free with Food*, one of the top one hundred cancer books of all time, faced her own daunting health challenge when she discovered a 3.7 cm tumor, of early stages of cancer in her lymphatic system. Growing up with Indigenous communities in the outback of Australia, Liana learned early on that simply cutting out a tumor without addressing its underlying causes could lead to its resurgence elsewhere in the body. This understanding resonated deeply with her, fueling her determination to delve deeper into her health rather than resort to the fear-driven route of surgery.

With courage, Liana intentionally sought out resources and experts to support her journey to heal. She says today that she discovered that an addiction to refined sugar and junk food was interfering in her ability to heal as a young woman. Through this process of introspection and change, her body dissolved the tumor within three months. Sixteen years later, she stands cancer-free, a testament to the power of trusting oneself and the body's innate ability to heal.

Her story underscores a crucial truth: You have to trust yourself more. No one can do the healing for you. True life transformation comes from within, from a deep understanding of our own bodies and experiences.

Cancer Is Not Random: It's a Wound-Healing Response

Cancer doesn't just show up one day like a thief in the night. It develops over time, and research is finally catching up to what some natural health practitioners have been saying for decades—cancer is part of the body's continual adaptation process, not a random genetic malfunction. Adaptation is required for survival and required for healing as our bodies encounter external forces in the form of physical, emotional, and chemical damage.

In a landmark paper, Harold F. Dvorak described tumors as "wounds that do not heal," a concept later expanded to show that cancer shares key pathways with embryonic development and tissue repair.[35] Dr. Max Gerson, MD, the founder of Gerson Therapy, said, "Cancer is not a disease in the sense most people think. It is a symptom, a final stage, that the body reaches after years of poisoning and nutritional deficiency. The tumor is not the problem—it is the body's solution to a deeper problem."[36]

Think of it this way: keep cutting the same spot on your hand and scar tissue forms. Ongoing toxins, chronic inflammation, or metabolic stress can trigger the same process inside the body. The body creates new growth as an attempt to repair and protect itself. Cancer is essentially a wound-healing process that does not turn off.

Research from Dr. Mina Bissell at Lawrence Berkeley National Laboratory supports this perspective. She demonstrated that cancerous cells placed in a healthy extracellular matrix would stop behaving like cancer. But when the environment remained toxic or inflamed, the cells continued to behave malignantly.[37]

So instead of asking, *how do we kill cancer?* We should be asking, why the cells are behaving this way and why the wound is still open.

If you want to understand why the wound is still open, and therefore cancer, you have to understand the difference between a healthy cell and a cancer cell. Once you see the contrast, the entire paradigm shifts. Cancer isn't some rogue invader, and it's not your body "going haywire." It's a biological adaptation to an unhealthy environment. Next, we will compare healthy cells and cancer cells to show that cancer growth can be an adaptive response, not a malfunction.

Healthy Cells: Order, Efficiency, and Cooperation

Healthy cells follow the rules, not because they are obedient, but because they operate within a structured intelligence.

- Healthy cells are structured, specialized, and integrated within tissues. They hold the form and function of the body together.
- They use oxygen-dependent energy production (oxidative phosphorylation) in the mitochondria, which is clean, efficient, and built for longevity.
- They listen to signals from the nervous system, hormones, and immune system, knowing when to grow, when to divide, and when to stop.

- When they are damaged or no longer needed, they undergo programmed cell death (apoptosis) because their role is to serve the body, not themselves.

Everything about a healthy cell is cooperative and efficient. When the environment changes and toxicity, inflammation, and metabolic stress build up, the body adapts to survive. That is when cancer cells step in.

Cancer Cells: Survival Mode in a Toxic Terrain
Cancer cells do not "break the rules"; they follow a different set of rules that helps them survive under extreme stress.

- **Rule 1:** Cancer cells lose their specialized structure and become free-moving, unstructured, and persistent. Why? Because if a cell is in a toxic, oxygen-deprived environment, it's better off being able to move, spread, and find nutrients wherever it can.
- **Rule 2:** Cancer cells often rely on fermentation, known as the Warburg effect, a simple sugar-burning process that works without oxygen. That is not a malfunction; it is a survival strategy. When oxygen is scarce and inflammation is high, cells either adapt or die. Cancer adapts.
- **Rule 3:** Instead of responding to normal growth signals, cancer cells start producing their own. They aren't listening to the body anymore because they are in survival mode.
- **Rule 4:** Cancer cells refuse to die. Why? Because the body's internal environment keeps signaling, "We are still in crisis." Cancer is just responding to that.

Cancer Isn't a Mistake. It Is the Body's Last Resort to Stay Alive.
This is where the mainstream paradigm gets it all wrong. The medical model tells you that cancer is a genetic accident, a random malfunction, a self-destructive disease. That narrative fuels fear and disempowerment. When you understand that cancer is a biological adaptation to a failing terrain, you start asking better questions.

- Instead of "How do we kill the cancer?" we should be asking, "What conditions in the body forced the cells to adapt this way?"
- Instead of "How do we cut it, poison it, or burn it?" we should be asking, "How do we make the body a place where cancer cells are no longer necessary?"

Cancer doesn't just show up out of nowhere. The body doesn't create disease without cause. Cancer cells appear because the body needs them to survive in the current conditions. Change the conditions, and the body no longer needs cancer. That is how you go from fighting cancer to understanding it so you can correct the cause.

Turbo Cancers and the COVID Shot

Something strange has been happening since 2021. Oncologists are seeing hyperaggressive cancers that seem to come out of nowhere. Tumors that should take years to grow are appearing within months.[38]

A study published in the journal *Cancers* (2023) found that repeated mRNA injections may contribute to immune exhaustion, particularly in T cell function, one of the immune system's primary defenses against cancer.[39] Dr. Angus Dalgleish, an oncologist in the UK, was one of the first to sound the alarm. He noticed an increase in turbo cancers following COVID-19 vaccination. His theory? The shots are dysregulating the immune system, impairing its ability to detect and suppress cancer cells.[40]

Others point to the role of spike proteins, lipid nanoparticles, and mRNA-induced inflammation as potential accelerators of oncogenesis.[41] The truth is, we don't yet have long-term studies. But we do have red flags.

Here's what we do know: immune dysregulation fuels cancer growth. If the body's surveillance system is impaired, cancer can take hold more easily. If inflammatory pathways are hijacked, tumor progression speeds up. And we've never before seen a global experiment with an mRNA platform that reprograms immune responses. Are we surprised that something seems off?

Cancer Is Not a Genetic Time Bomb

For decades, we've been told cancer is genetic: bad luck, bad DNA, or an unavoidable hereditary curse. That narrative is largely false.

The *Journal of the National Cancer Institute* states that only 5–10 percent of cancers are truly genetic.[42] The rest? Environmental, metabolic, and lifestyle-driven. Cancer is not a disease of bad genes; rather, it is a disease of a bad environment, such as:

- Toxins—Pesticides, plastics, heavy metals, EMFs, and endocrine disruptors are everywhere.
- Diet—Ultra-processed foods, seed oils, and sugar-fueled metabolic dysfunction create an internal breeding ground for cancer.
- Chronic Stress—Dysregulation of the nervous system suppresses immune function, paving the way for tumor growth.[43]

As we talked about in the last chapter, if genes determined everything, identical twins would get cancer at the same rate. They don't. How you live trumps genetics nearly every time.

The Myth of "Early Detection Saves Lives"

We've all heard the mantra: "Early detection saves lives." It's been drilled into us by countless public health campaigns, urging regular screenings for various cancers. But what if this well-intentioned advice isn't the universal truth it's made out to be? What if, in most cases, early detection doesn't significantly extend life and might even lead to unnecessary interventions?

A comprehensive study published on August 28, 2023, titled "Estimated Lifetime Gained with Cancer Screening Tests," examined the effectiveness of several common cancer screenings. This study followed 2.1 million individuals over an average of ten to fifteen years, comparing those who underwent screenings to those who did not.[44] The screenings evaluated included:

- Mammography for breast cancer
- Colonoscopy, sigmoidoscopy, or fecal occult blood testing (FOBT) for colorectal cancer
- Computed tomography (CT) for lung cancer
- Prostate-specific antigen (PSA) testing for prostate cancer

Findings:
No significant difference in lifetime gained was observed for:

- Mammography
- PSA testing
- Colonoscopy
- Annual or biennial FOBT
- CT scans for lung cancer

Only sigmoidoscopy showed a meaningful benefit. This exam of the lower large intestine was linked to an average lifetime gain of about 110 days from screening. These findings challenge the blanket assertion that all cancer screenings unequivocally save lives.[45]

The Problem of Overdiagnosis

One of the critical issues with widespread screening is overdiagnosis, the detection of cancers that would not have caused problems during a person's lifetime. This can lead to overtreatment, exposing individuals to the risks and side effects of interventions without a clear benefit.

For instance, a significant increase in thyroid cancer diagnoses has been observed in South Korea, primarily due to the introduction of widespread ultrasonography screening. However, this surge in detection did not correspond to a rise in mortality rates, suggesting that many of these cancers were not life-threatening.[46]

Similarly, prostate cancer screenings using the PSA test have been debated due to the potential for overdiagnosis. Many detected prostate cancers grow so slowly that they would not pose a significant threat during a man's lifetime. Yet, the diagnosis often leads to treatments that can cause incontinence, impotence, and other serious side effects.[47]

Some conditions that are now labeled "cancer" used to be considered benign, nonthreatening and acknowledged as things that would self-resolve. A notable example is ductal carcinoma in situ (DCIS), which is a noninvasive form of breast cancer that may never progress but is often treated aggressively.[48]

The conversation around cancer is riddled with misunderstandings—we fear tumors without questioning why they form, and we chase early detection without asking if it truly saves lives. But cancer isn't the only condition where the mainstream narrative falls apart.

Autoimmunity: Not the Body Attacking Itself

Autoimmune diseases are rising at an alarming rate, and just like cancer, they are widely misunderstood.[49] The conventional model paints autoimmunity as the body turning against itself, a tragic case of self-destruction. Doctors tell patients their immune system is "malfunctioning," randomly attacking the thyroid, joints, nervous system, or skin. The message is clear: your body is broken, and your immune system has lost its ability to recognize friend from foe. But is that really what's happening?

Or is the immune system, like cancer cells, responding to a deeper problem, trying to adapt to a failing environment? The immune system doesn't attack for no reason.

If you cut your finger, what happens? The immune system rushes in to heal it. White blood cells surround the wound, inflammation increases, and new tissue starts to form. This isn't random destruction; it is repair.

Now apply that same logic to autoimmunity. The immune system doesn't start attacking tissue without a trigger. It is not a rogue assassin; it is a surveillance system. When it targets the thyroid (Hashimoto's), the joints (rheumatoid arthritis), or the gut (Crohn's), it is not a mistake; it is an effort to clear something out.

The real question isn't *why is the immune system attacking?* What is it trying to get rid of?

The Root Causes of Autoimmunity

Autoimmune disease rates have exploded in the last few decades, and it's not because human biology suddenly changed. Most autoimmune conditions do not appear out of nowhere. They follow a pattern: years of chronic inflammation, toxic exposures, infections, or metabolic dysfunction often come before the diagnosis. The immune system is reacting to something, and when we look deeper, we often find:[50]

- Leaky gut—When the gut barrier breaks down due to processed foods, glyphosate exposure, and chronic stress, food particles and toxins enter the bloodstream. The immune system reacts as if it's under attack, launching chronic inflammation that never turns off.[51]

- Chronic infections—Viruses like Epstein-Barr, Lyme bacteria, and other stealth pathogens don't always go away. Instead, they persist at low levels, keeping the immune system in constant overdrive. A hyperactive immune system does not mean it is malfunctioning; it means it is fighting an ongoing battle against a threat it recognizes.[52]

- Toxins—Heavy metals like mercury, pesticide residues like glyphosate, and mold toxins all disrupt immune signaling. When toxins build up, the body works to neutralize them—but in doing so, it can trigger autoimmune responses.[53]

- Artificial immune stimulation—Perhaps the most overlooked culprit is the modern vaccine schedule. Instead of allowing immunity to mature through ordinary exposures, it relies on designed immune triggers and adjuvants such as aluminum salts to boost the response. Some researchers and clinicians question whether this can unsettle immune balance, though public health authorities consider the schedule safe and effective.[54]

Consider this: Since the early 1990s, the childhood vaccine schedule has roughly tripled, and diagnoses of autoimmune disorders have risen over the same period, including rheumatoid arthritis, type 1 diabetes, lupus, and multiple sclerosis.[55] Is this just a coincidence? The immune system isn't designed to be forcefully hijacked over and over again. This hyperstimulation leads to immune confusion, where the body no longer recognizes self from invader.

The very industry that claims to be "protecting" the immune system may be the one breaking it. Instead of suppressing the immune system with drugs, we should be asking: what is the immune system fighting, and how do we remove the root cause?

Hashimoto's: The Perfect Example

Take Hashimoto's thyroiditis, one of the most common autoimmune diseases today. The standard explanation? *The immune system is attacking the thyroid.* But why? Is it actually targeting the thyroid itself, or is it trying to eliminate something harmful inside the tissue?

Many Hashimoto's patients test positive for:

- Viral reactivations (like Epstein-Barr virus)[56]
- High levels of environmental toxins (pesticides, heavy metals)[57]
- Inflammatory food triggers (like gluten and dairy, which mimic thyroid tissue proteins)[58]

The immune system is acting as designed and responding to perceived threats. When years of stress, infection, or toxicity damage the thyroid, the immune system steps in to repair. That is not an error. It is an adaptation.

The Future: Restore the Terrain, Stop the War

The old model of attack and suppression is failing. It does not work. The new model is to support the body's healing capacity.

Cancer and autoimmunity are not mistakes; they are survival strategies pushed beyond their purpose. The goal is not to fight the body but to restore balance by meeting its needs.

That means:

- Fix the terrain. Clean food, clean water, detox pathways open.
- Heal metabolism. Cancer thrives on glucose. The right diet starves it.
- Balance the nervous system. Chronic stress, trauma, and dysregulated fight-or-flight responses weaken immune function and fuel disease.
- Remove toxins. No more bombarding the body with carcinogens.
- Build the immune system. Not suppress it, but train it to work right.

The body is the best doctor you have. It's time to stop fighting it and start working with it.

The Shift from Treatment to Healing, Even with Cancer

A dear friend of ours was diagnosed with an aggressive cancer that ultimately took her life. What made it even more heartbreaking was that she found the very knowledge she had been searching for, just a little too late.

In her final weeks, she discovered the vitalistic principles that so many never hear about: the body's innate intelligence, its ability to heal, and the power of aligning with nature instead of fighting against it. I'll never forget the phone call. With wonder in her voice, she asked, "Is it true? Could healing really be this simple?" She was talking about the nervous system and how shifting from fight-or-flight into rest and repair can unlock healing potential she was never told about.

Even in the face of death, she came alive. Her curiosity returned, her excitement bubbled over like a child discovering something wonderful for the first time. It was incredible to witness. She dove into this new paradigm with joy, not regret. She felt peace, finally, because she had found truth.

Her journey reminds us just how critical it is to understand how healing actually happens.

For five years, she fought valiantly. She lost fifty pounds. She hand-ground apricot seeds. She spent thousands on the best integrative treatments. She took every supplement, used the machines, ate only pure, whole foods and herbs. She was faithful, unwavering, and never seduced by the false promises of the cancer industry. She didn't fear death. But she was searching for something more, something that made sense.

Nine weeks before she passed, she found it. Vitalism. The body's design. The missing piece.

"I can't wait to get home and switch all of my kids to this kind of care," she told us. Even as her time here was running out, she was thinking about her children's future. She didn't just want them to survive; she wanted them to thrive, guided by truth.

Her story is a sacred reminder: **matter has limits**. Healing is possible, but timing matters. Sometimes, the interference has gone too far, the body too depleted. That's why we can't wait for a diagnosis or a breaking point. We need to align with the laws of life now, before crisis arrives.

Let her story be the wake-up call we all need. Start before it's too late.

Don't wait for symptoms to give you permission. Vitalism isn't an alternative; it's the foundation of life and health. Embracing it is more than a hopeful idea. It is the difference between chasing symptoms, "naturally" or conventionally, and truly living.

* * *

Your body isn't broken. It's communicating. Are you willing to listen and make a change? Part 1 was about seeing through the false promises of Medicine and exposing the necessity to exit conventional Medicine to heal. Part 2 is about rediscovering what it means to truly *live*. Cancer and autoimmunity reveal the devastating effects of a body pushed to its extremes to adapt, but they also point us toward the solution: restoring vitality.

In the next section, we'll move into living naturally by uncovering nature's laws of healing and exposing the top things that interfere with healing in the twenty-first century. From toxic beliefs to toxic foods, from movement to microbiomes, from structure to stress, we'll uncover the hidden interferences that keep you stuck in survival mode and the simple, powerful shifts that return you to a state of resilience.

PART II

Live Naturally

Principle 1: Your body was designed to heal.
Principle 2: **The Body Can Become Devitalized.**

You'll recall the first principle is "Your body was designed to heal." The body can also be depleted. Devitalization happens when the laws of biology are broken long enough to cause disruption. Toxic inputs, chronic stress, nutrient-depleted food, nervous system interference, and lack of proper movement and breathing aren't just irrtants. They suppress the body's ability to repair, adapt, and thrive. Over time, matter adapts to a lower state of vitality. It's called devitalization, and it's what ultimately leads to disease.

It's the reality of living out of rhythm with how the body was created to function. But the same system that adapts downward can adapt back, if you remove the interference(s). Most people don't need to add more to their lives, they need to remove what's in the way.

Living naturally means aligning with how your body was created to thrive. It means turning away from synthetic inputs and returning to real food, real movement, real rest, and real connection. It's about building resilience, not adding restrictions.

In the chapters ahead, we'll break down what this looks like in real life. You'll learn how to identify and eliminate the interferences that are blocking your body from healing: gut dysfunction, toxic thoughts, processed food, chemical overload, spinal misalignment. This is how you reclaim the vitality you were designed for.

CHAPTER 7

The Cause Is the Cure

The only cure is getting to the cause.
—Dr. Charles Majors

I was once asked, "Do you think there's a cure for cancer that's being hidden?"

Here's the truth: we're not going to find the cure to cancer, or any chronic disease, in a pill. Not now. Not ever. And despite what some in the natural health world believe, the cure isn't hidden in a remote jungle or locked away by Big Pharma. That idea might make for a compelling headline or help sell the latest berry-based supplement, but it misses the point.

You need to identify what is interfering with your body's ability to function and heal. That is the missing link in most care models. It is not a matter of adding more. It is a matter of removing what is in the way. This is what we call "The Interference Equation." And there are three main categories to look for: **Thoughts, traumas, toxins.**

These are the three Ts that devitalize the body. They block adaptation. They drain your reserves. They create miscommunication between systems, and they eventually lead to dysfunction, then disease. When you remove them, the body responds. When you leave them unaddressed, the body adapts to a lower state of vitality.

You Were Built to Adapt
The brilliance of the human body is in its ability to adapt. It heals, rebuilds, and recalibrates in real time. You cut your skin and it heals. You get a virus

and your body produces antibodies. You fast and your body starts breaking down diseased tissue for fuel. These are not accidents. This is a system that is responsive and intelligent.

But even the most intelligent system can be overwhelmed. Healing is possible in the right conditions, not all conditions. If the body is constantly assaulted by stress, chemical irritants, poor sleep, unresolved injuries, and unrelenting demands, it will eventually stop adapting upward and start adapting downward. That is the beginning of devitalization.

Most people do not feel this shift all at once. It is subtle. You go from waking up refreshed to waking up groggy. From sleeping through the night to tossing and turning. From bouncing back from illness to lingering fatigue that never fully lifts. From a sharp, focused mind to brain fog and forgetfulness.

You do not go from vital to broken overnight. You go from vibrant to tired to wired to sick. You go from adapting to surviving.

The 3 Ts: What They Are and How They Interfere

1. Thoughts: The Mental Loop That Rewrites Your Physiology
Thoughts are not just private ideas. They are physiological events. Every thought sends a cascade of electrical and chemical signals through the body.[1] Chronic fear, resentment, hopelessness, and even busyness wire your nervous system for survival, not healing.[2]

When your mind rehearses stress, your body produces cortisol. When you ruminate on worst-case scenarios, your immune system slows down. When your identity is built on achievement, your adrenals do not get a break.

The sympathetic nervous system, your fight-or-flight mode, is essential for moments of danger. But most people are stuck there by default.[3] Over time, the body cannot keep up. The gut becomes inflamed. Hormones become imbalanced. Sleep becomes shallow. Energy tanks. And because it is mental, it is often overlooked.

One of the most dangerous lies in health today is this: "If I just do all the right things, I'll get better."

No, not if your nervous system is stuck in fight-or-flight mode because of your thought-life. You can be the healthiest person in the world on paper and still be devitalized. Because your thoughts shape your biology.[4]

2. Traumas: Physical Stress That Disconnects the Brain and Body

We live in a physical world. Your body carries memory in its structure. Injuries, poor posture, birth trauma, sports accidents, falls, and surgeries can create long-term disruptions in the spine and nervous system. The spine is not just a stack of bones; it is the protective housing for your spinal cord, the highway of communication between the brain and the body.

When that communication is blocked or distorted, the organs and systems it controls suffer. Blood pressure rises. Digestion weakens. Respiration alters. Inflammation increases.

Modern life creates the perfect environment for trauma-based interference. We sit for hours, bend our heads forward over screens, live in shoes that compromise our foundation, and move far less than we were designed to.

These physical stresses do not always cause pain, but they always create compensation. The nervous system reroutes, the muscles adapt, the joints degenerate, and before long you are living in a body that feels foreign and fragile. This is structural devitalization.

Correcting this requires more than stretching. It requires realignment of the spine, movement patterns, and the nervous system.

3. Toxins: The Chemical Assault on Vitality

We are being poisoned slowly.

The water has microplastics. The air has endocrine disruptors. The food has seed oils, pesticides, artificial flavors, and preservatives that your grandparents would not even recognize as food. And the medications meant to treat symptoms come with side effects that wreck your liver, microbiome, and mood.

Toxins do not just make you feel off. They hijack your cell receptors. They mimic hormones. They overwhelm your detox systems. And they create inflammation at the cellular level that blocks healing responses from ever initiating.

The body is designed to detoxify. Your liver, lymph, gut, and skin are constantly working to eliminate waste. But when the input exceeds the capacity, the result is overload. Your body begins to store what it cannot eliminate.

This is why cleansing is not a trend. It is a necessity.

The Sum of the Load

It is tempting to look for a single cause of disease. One nutrient deficiency. One infection. One diagnosis. But the reality is that disease is almost always the result of cumulative interference.

A little stress, a little misalignment, a few skipped nights of sleep, a few rounds of antibiotics, a few decades of processed food. The body keeps the score, and the result is not just symptoms. It is a system stuck in defense, unable to shift into repair.

This is the vitality equation no one is talking about: **Vitality = Design – Interference**

If the body was designed to heal, then healing will happen when interference is removed.

Healing Is a Subtraction Equation

In biology, healing happens when you create space for it. Lake Erie healed when industrial toxins were removed.[5] Barren farmland regenerates when big-scale commercial farming practices are replaced with proper stewardship of the land.[6] But most people have been trained to believe they need to add more. More labs. More protocols. More workouts. More pills.

But ask yourself this: What if the body is not broken? What if it is blocked? What if you are not tired because of aging, but because you are burning all your energy trying to survive an environment you were not designed for?

What if your anxiety is not a chemical imbalance, but a by-product of a life stuck in high alert mode? What if your immune issues are not bad luck, but a signal that your body has been sounding the alarm for years, and no one has been listening?

Healing begins when you stop getting in the way. This is the radical shift. We are not adding a cure. We are removing the interference. We are restoring alignment to a system that wants to heal.

And in the next section of the book, you'll learn how to assess it. You'll identify the thoughts, traumas, and toxins that are draining you, and the habits, rhythms, and environments that are building you up. We call it your "Vitality Balance Sheet." Just like a financial audit reveals cash flow problems, this audit will show you what's devitalizing you and what's restoring you. You'll use it as your compass, because you can't rebuild what you haven't accounted for.

But for now, just remember this: if your health isn't where you want it to be, it's not because your body forgot how to heal. It's because something is in the way.

What Interference Looks Like in Real Life

Interference does not always show up in lab results. It shows up in daily life. You need coffee to wake up and something else to fall asleep. That is interference.

You eat clean but still get bloated. That is interference.

You get headaches at 3 p.m. You snap at your kids. You feel tired but wired. You dread social events. You cannot think straight when you skip a meal. You crash after workouts. That is interference. And it is not just physical. It is emotional and neurological. But the body knows how to recalibrate. You just have to give it the chance.

From Chronic Fatigue to Vitality

Stephanie was a single mom of two. What started as exhaustion soon turned into chronic fatigue, body-wide pain, and an almost constant sensitivity to touch. Medicine labeled it as fibromyalgia. But labels like that often become a way of saying, "This is your new normal."

She knew this couldn't be her normal. Medications didn't help. They masked some of the symptoms temporarily, but she could feel herself fading. She fell asleep next to her kids because she was too exhausted to transition to her own bed.

Stephanie's body wasn't broken. It was responding to years of a nervous system that was wildly out of balance. What she needed wasn't a new diagnosis. She needed a reset. When we helped her address the three Ts—thoughts, traumas, and toxins—her nervous system recalibrated. The pain lifted. The fatigue lifted. Her body healed. She didn't just get better. She got her life back.

The Body Is Not Your Enemy

There is a reason this chapter matters so much. Because most people do not just suffer physically. They begin to believe that something is wrong with them. They turn against their own body.

But your body is not sabotaging you. It is adapting to what it has been given. Your symptoms are not failures. They are feedback. You were not born defective. You were born into a world that has trained you to ignore your design and override your instincts. And now it is time to come back to center.

This is the pivot point. In the chapters ahead, we will begin removing the three Ts and restoring what your body has been begging for. You will learn how to reset your nervous system, cleanse your internal environment, nourish your biology, and reconnect with the physical rhythms of breath, movement, and rest.

Because you do not need a better protocol. You need a better foundation. And the foundation begins here: remove the interference, and vitality returns.

CHAPTER 8

Primary Toxicity:
The Dark Side of Belief

Fear is the path to the dark side. Fear leads to anger. Anger leads to hate. Hate leads to suffering.

—Yoda

We live in a world obsessed with external threats: food dyes, artificial colors, industrial chemicals, electromagnetic frequencies, etc. But what if the most overlooked toxin isn't something you ingest or inhale . . . it's something you believe? The thoughts you rehearse daily, the identity you accept, and the fears you carry aren't abstract. They shape your body. They rewire your brain. They dictate your healing potential.

Toxic Thoughts, Real Damage
People often use the terms "mind" and "brain" interchangeably. But the brain is the hardware. The mind is the software and it's in charge. Dr. Caroline Leaf says it plainly: "Your body is not in control of your mind—your mind is in control of your body."[1]

Studies show that 75–98 percent of physical, mental, and behavioral illnesses come from thought life.[2] The way you think affects your immune system, digestion, hormones, and pain thresholds. Emotions can speed up or stall healing.[3]

One study even showed that people experiencing chronic frustration, anger, and fear had DNA that coiled more tightly, reducing the expression of certain genes tied to healing and cellular repair. But when those same people shifted into feelings of love, gratitude, and appreciation, their DNA relaxed, and those healing genes were reactivated.[4] This is a measurable, biological, and a life-changing truth of epigenetics that we explored earlier.

The Poisoned Mind

Let's talk about sham knee surgery.

In a 2002 *New England Journal of Medicine* study, world-renowned surgeon Dr. Bruce Moseley operated on two groups of patients with knee arthritis. One group got the real procedure. The other got "sham" surgery: numbing injection, water splashed for sound effects, stitches for show but no real procedure.[5] Get this! One third of the sham group reported complete resolution of their knee pain, which was the same rate of success as the surgery group. At one point in the observations, the placebo group had better outcomes. That's the power of belief.

There's also a psychiatric case of a woman with multiple personalities. In one personality, she was diabetic. In the other, she wasn't. Her blood sugar levels literally changed based on who she believed she was at that moment.[6]

Most are familiar with the placebo effect, and the sham knee surgery is a clear example of it. But the opposite also exists. Remember the *nocebo effect*?

In a startling experiment published in *The Pavlovian Journal of Biological Science* (1981), thirty-four unsuspecting college students were connected to electrodes and told a mild electric current would pass through their heads. They were warned it might produce symptoms like headaches or tingling. But here's the kicker: **no current was ever applied.** Yet, over two-thirds reported headaches, sometimes accompanied by extreme tension or discomfort.[7] The researchers concluded that focusing on pain, even in clinical settings, can amplify or even create it. In their words: "Clinical focusing on pain may itself be a cause of pain"

One study showed that women who believed they were prone to heart disease were four times more likely to die of it, even though their diet, blood pressure, cholesterol, and family history were no worse than anyone else's.[8] The only measurable difference was belief.

Another study found that nearly half of asthma patients experienced relief from a fake inhaler or sham acupuncture.[9]

- Forty percent of those with headaches improved with a sugar pill.[10]
- Half of colitis patients experienced complete remission after being given a placebo.[11]
- Forty percent of those struggling with infertility got pregnant while taking fake fertility drugs.[12]
- For pain, placebos often outperform morphine.[13]
- For anxiety and depression, *nearly all the positive* effects of antidepressants may come from placebo.[14] One study showed that when the same drug was given but described as something unrelated to mood, patients reported no improvement in their emotions.[15]

When you believe something harmful will happen, your body responds, whether real or not.

Clear the Path

Eric Kandel, a Nobel Prize–winning neuropsychiatrist, showed that even our imaginations can affect gene expression, turning certain genes on or off depending on our thoughts.[16] This means your brain isn't hardwired. It's live-wired. You are not a victim of your biology. Your biology is a victim of your neurology.

Imagine you're in a dense forest. You start cutting a path. That path didn't exist before, but now it does. The more you walk it, the more permanent it becomes. Stop using it, and the forest overtakes it. Your brain works the same way. Every thought, every emotion, every repeated experience becomes a path, a neural circuit etched into your physical brain.

That's why negative patterns and self-limiting beliefs feel so hard to break. They became traumas to your mind, and your brain wired these traumas into your nervous system. But here's the good news: even if your brain has been shaped by dysfunction, it's not a death sentence. You can build new paths, access those new paths over and over, and eventually the old, unused paths are no longer accessed.[17]

You've most likely noticed that I write more directly from a Christian worldview. This will be especially present in the mindset parts of the book. Not to exclude anyone, but when it comes to the battle for the mind, I've found the Bible offers unmatched insight and real solutions.

Even if you don't share my biblical beliefs, I invite you to examine the time-tested wisdom and neurobiological truth that can change your life. If you're willing to engage, maybe even wrestle, with what's presented, I believe you'll come away stronger.

Young men and women raised in poverty, addiction, and violence have turned their lives around. They've graduated from college, raised families, and led their communities. Why? Because they changed how they think, and the brain followed.[18]

Renew the Mind

Romans 12:2 says, *Do not conform to the pattern of this world, but be transformed by the renewing of your mind.*

Transformed. That word jumps off the page. In Greek, the word Paul, the writer of Romans from the Bible, uses is metamorphoō, the root of our English word "metamorphosis." It's the same word used to describe Jesus's transfiguration in the Gospels. This isn't about polishing up your mindset. It's not a mental tune-up. Like a caterpillar becoming a butterfly, it's a total change in form and function.

The word for "renewing" is anakainōsis, from *ana-* ("again" or "up") and *kainos* ("new in kind, unprecedented"). It doesn't mean recycling old thoughts. It means something entirely new is being built within you. A complete renovation.

But notice what the author didn't say. He didn't say you'd be transformed by changing your circumstances. Or by finding the right doctor. Or by finally getting the diagnosis. He said transformation begins by renewing your mind. So what does that actually mean?

Renewing the mind isn't just thinking positive thoughts. It's the daily process of choosing truth over lies. It's replacing fear-based narratives with faith-rooted convictions. It's choosing not to conform to the world's cynicism, medical labels, and generational patterns, and instead to rewire your mind around what God says is true. It's intentional, active, and sacred. Just like a house under renovation, parts of your mind need to be stripped, rebuilt, and restored. Some beliefs need demolition. Others need reinforcement. That's the work of renewal.

And it's not a one-time event. It's daily. Sometimes hourly. We'll walk through specific strategies for renewing your mind later in this book. But for now, here's the truth I want you to settle: your healing doesn't start in your bloodwork. It starts in your beliefs. If you want transformation in your health, it starts between your ears and into your thoughts and beliefs.

Hope Is a Biological Force

Take one of my favorite stories, an experiment from Johns Hopkins scientist Curt Paul Richter.

He placed rats in buckets of high water. On average, they swam around for fifteen minutes, gave up, and drowned. But when he rescued a rat just before it sank, dried it off, then put it back in the water . . . that same rat swam for sixty hours. That's 240 times longer.[19] What changed? Hope. The rat believed rescue was possible.

We are taught to put limits on what the body can do. But the reality is, we don't fully know the healing potential of the body. When you change your thoughts, you change your physiology. And when you maintain hope, you activate something far more powerful than any medication: your will to live.

The Lie of "False Hope"

At this point, you might wonder, *What if I get my hopes up, only to be let down?*

That's the fear of disappointment talking. And it's understandable, especially for those who've been sick for years, gone from doctor to doctor, or watched someone they love suffer. But here's the truth: there's no such thing as false hope when your hope is rightly placed.

False hope is what happens when you put your trust in the therapy, the pill, the procedure. And yes, those things can fail you. But hope rooted in truth, in faith, in the divinely designed resilience of your body is not false. It's foundational.

Faith doesn't guarantee the outcome. But it guarantees transformation in the process. When you hope rightly, you're defying limitations. That's what the rescued rat did. That's what the patients in the sham surgery group did. That's what you're called to do: refuse to conform to the pattern of fear and despair, and instead *renew your mind* around what is eternally true.

The real risk isn't in hoping too much. The real risk is letting fear shrink your life before disease ever does. Hope isn't dangerous. Hopelessness is.

Giving someone false promises isn't hope; it's lying. Real hope isn't what you tell other people. It's what you tell yourself. It's the agreement between you and your Creator that your body is not broken, your life is not random, and your story is not over.

Late-Stage Cancer

I think of David here. He was diagnosed with late-stage prostate cancer. After a full battery of tests, the doctors sat across from him and said, "Even with aggressive treatment, it's very likely this will return." He could have accepted that as his fate. Many would have. But David didn't.

Instead, he made a decision: *"I'm going all in on health. Not fear. Not waiting. Not managing. I'm going after it."*

He fasted. He cleansed. He aligned his spine. He detoxed his thoughts as much as his body. And he stayed fiercely committed—removing interference in every form. That meant rejecting the idea that the cancer was in control. It meant rejecting the timeline he was handed.

And David healed. It's been eight years as of this writing. He didn't just survive. He transformed. He now references his cancer journey as the catalyst for change.

I've seen it a lot over the years. I no longer call it *remission*. That's a medical word that implies a potential comeback, like something bad is lurking in the shadows. Why would we use language that gives power to disease? It puts you in the passenger seat. David chose to drive.

You Are Not a Victim

This is where the vitalistic philosophy separates itself. We believe the body is designed brilliantly. We trust its resilience. We focus on restoring function, not chasing diagnosis codes. And ultimately, we believe that we were not given the spirit of fear but of power, love, and sound mind (2 Timothy 1:7). Fear doesn't fit there. Wisdom inhabits that space, divine guidance and well-timed principled solutions.

You are not a statistic. You are not a diagnosis. You are not a label. You are not a victim of biology or circumstance. You are a living testimony that the mind, renewed by truth, can change everything.

This is what's missing in today's clinical model: empowerment. Medicine is not the enemy. Medicine is doing the best it can with the two tools it has: drugs and surgery. But knowing what we know about how powerful the mind is, why aren't we pouring time, energy, and resources into educating and equipping people to take ownership over their mind and health? And why on Earth do we tolerate the foretelling of our future based on genes (not based on genetic expression but simple genetic predisposition) and medical rates of success?

You say, "that's what psychiatry is for." But nine times out of ten, people leave that office with a prescription, not a blueprint for governing their thoughts. We need more than labels and medication. We need ownership. We need people to reclaim their God-given agency.

So, if a renewed mind sounds like the key to unlocking healing and vitality, you aren't wrong. But stopping there would ignore one of your nervous system's most vital biological requirements: movement and breath. Not just workouts. Not even exercise as you know it. In the next chapter, we'll uncover why your body may not be moving the way you want and why laziness isn't to blame, it's a biological signal that your nervous system craves something more.

CHAPTER 9

Sedentary Is a Symptom

Strong people are harder to kill than weak people, and more useful in general.

—Mark Rippetoe

You weren't born tired. You were born to move. So why does it feel so hard just to get up and go? Why does a simple walk feel like a full workout, and a real workout feel impossible?

This isn't because of laziness. It's also not simply a lack of discipline or motivation. It's often a system-wide shutdown. Your body is not resisting movement out of defiance; it is protecting you from what it perceives as unsafe.

Most people blame themselves. But sedentary behavior is often the most overlooked symptom of a nervous system stuck in defense, a body flooded with stress chemistry, and alignment patterns that make movement feel dangerous.[1] In other words, if you're not moving, it might be because your body is trying to survive.

Nervous System in Lockdown

When your nervous system senses danger, performance is not the priority, protection is. Movement gets shut down. Muscles brace. Initiative fades. You stop engaging with the world because your system doesn't feel safe in it. It becomes more than a mindset problem but rather an ingrained biological pattern. And it gets worse.

When physical, mental, or chemical stress becomes chronic, your biochemistry breaks down. Chronic stress depletes cellular energy. Your mitochondria, the power plants inside your cells, stop producing energy efficiently. Your cells literally generate less adenosine triphosphate (ATP), the fuel needed for movement.[2] When ATP drops, your body gets sluggish, heavy, inflamed. You don't avoid movement because you're lazy. Your body might be signaling that it can't afford to move. It's conserving energy to survive. And "powering through" that conservation is a losing and unwise endeavor.

Movement as Medicine

Movement is how your body heals. It pumps lymph, a clear fluid that moves through your body to remove waste, fight infection, and carry out immune cells. Movement regulates hormones. It supports detoxification. It activates the brain. Without it, these systems get congested. Lymph stagnates. Hormones misfire. And detox pathways back up.

Your brain has its own waste-removal system, the glymphatic system, which clears toxins and metabolic waste during states of rest and rhythm.[3] It relies on fluid movement through brain tissue and functions best when your nervous system is regulated, your posture is aligned, and your breathing is deep and steady.

Without this rhythmic clearance, waste builds up and brain function suffers. This is why movement is essential. It's not aesthetics. It's function. Motion is the signal that tells your body it's safe to repair.

Conditioned for Weakness

Everything around you trains you to be passive. Sit through school. Sit at your desk. Sit on the couch to relax. Modern life was built for convenience, not vitality. You weren't made for this environment, and the longer you live in it, the more unnatural it feels to move. Your innate craving for movement becomes dull as your nervous system is out of balance.

If you've ever seen the movie *WALL-E*, you know what I'm talking about. The humans are so used to being passive that when they fall out of their chairs, they literally can't stand back up. It was satire. But now it's starting to feel like a prophecy. There is a global shift toward engineered dependence. The weaker and sicker people are, the easier they are to manage. Without muscle, there is no resistance. Without energy, there is no uprising. Without movement, there is no freedom.

Just Move.

I've been doing this long enough to know that simply telling you that movement is good for you and that you should do it won't move the needle. I also know that we've been conditioned to overthink everything, especially when it comes to movement. We analyze. We hesitate. We try to "understand" our way to action. You hear things like "you shouldn't start exercising without getting advice from a doctor" or "don't start until you feel better."

Sometimes, the answer isn't more information. It's motion. You now know that sedentary behavior often stems from neurological, metabolic, or structural interference. But this is where most people get stuck. Instead of decoding the signal, they start to identify with it.

"I'm in sympathetic dominance."

"My body's too inflamed."

"I'm too stressed."

And just like that, the nervous system cements a pattern of passivity. Not because you're lazy. Because you've been *living in lockdown.* But the nervous system doesn't shift through awareness alone. It changes through behavior. You can't think your way out of a dysregulated state. You have to *move* your way out.

The longer you stay inactive, the more that circuitry becomes default. Over time, you're not just tired, you're *trained* to be tired.

Story: Rachel and the Fifteen-Minute Reset

I had a patient, Rachel, who was in her mid-thirties, hadn't exercised in over five years and had massive anxiety around the idea of "exercise." Her hormones were off, her sleep was inconsistent, and her motivation was zero. Movement is essential to balancing hormones and impacting sleep. She thought she needed a full workout plan, a trainer, and a perfect diet. Because of this belief, she didn't take action for months.

So we started with one simple thing: sunwalks. Fifteen minutes. Every morning. Just movement and light.

Three weeks later, she was sleeping better. Fewer headaches. More energy. Not because she was crushing high-intensity workouts. But because her nervous system finally felt safe to turn back on.

Sunwalking: The Nervous System Reboot

When you move your body while exposing your eyes to natural light, you reset your circadian rhythm, boost serotonin, and signal to your brain: *engage.* Morning sunlight through your eyes also raises cortisol *at the right time.*[4]

Quick note—**skip the sunglasses**. When light hits your eyes directly, it stimulates specialized cells in the retina called intrinsically photosensitive retinal ganglion cells (ipRGCs). These are the messengers to your brain's internal clock. They don't work the same through tinted lenses. Direct morning light into your eyes (never staring at the sun, but eyes open to the sky) anchors your circadian rhythm and boosts mental clarity, hormone balance, and sleep quality.[3]

That's right, cortisol is not your enemy. It just needs to show up at the right time. When it rises naturally in the morning (thanks to sun exposure and movement), it sets your internal clock and helps you fall asleep at night. Pair sunwalking with slow, nasal breathing and steady rhythm, and you've got a built-in neurological reset.

It's not complicated. It's how your biology was designed to function. Walk toward the sun. Breathe through your nose. Let your system recalibrate. That's where it starts. Walking is rhythmic. It's bilateral. It's grounding. It doesn't spike cortisol. It reengages your vestibular system, your breath, your posture.

If you feel stuck, fatigued, or dysregulated, this is a reset button. It's not glamorous. But it works. Walk until movement feels normal again.

Push Until It's Patterned

Now, let's talk about the other side of the equation and the fitness lie: powering through. The fitness industry sold us the idea that more intensity equals better results. As a former personal trainer, I know this firsthand because I both studied it and taught it to clients.

I used to teach high-intensity interval training. That you have to crush yourself to get fit. And it worked for a season. But I now believe that high intensity is not what most people need. For most people, it's gasoline on a nervous system already on fire.

When your nervous system is dysregulated, intense workouts often do more harm than good. They reinforce stress patterns. They spike cortisol. They tax already depleted reserves.

There's a difference between being "soft" and being wise. If you've been consistently moving your body or if fitness is part of your lifestyle, your nervous system is already wired for that rhythm. You don't have to second-guess whether today is a rest day or a walk day. You've built the reps, and your body knows what's safe.

But if you're not in that rhythm yet, don't confuse "listening to your body" with obeying your comfy. Your body doesn't want comfort. It wants consistency. If you've been living in sedentary mode, your "intuition" might lie to you. Not because it's broken, but because it's trained by a broken routine.

So if you are needing more movement, it will take getting uncomfortable and breaking what "feels right" to get into a healthy pattern of fueling your cells with oxygen, strengthening your frame and lungs, detoxing, supporting lymphatic flow and training your mind to break barriers.

Now, let's make a distinction. The nervous system needs rest. Rest is sacred. We are designed to have breaks and have periods of stillness. To rest, meditate, and pray. But sedentary living, the kind that numbs your biology and disconnects you from your physical body, that's dysfunction not peace.

Breath: The Missing Link for Motion

When you're stuck in stress mode, even breathing becomes dysfunctional and movement seems exhausting. Shallow, chest-driven breaths send danger signals to the brain, keeping your nervous system in a low-grade fight-or-flight loop. It's a biological lockdown that makes stillness feel like survival and movement feel unsafe.

If you're not breathing deeply, your body won't feel safe enough to move freely. That's why so many people struggle to *start*. Their nervous system isn't waiting on motivation; it's waiting on oxygen. Intentional breath resets your internal state for safety. Studies show that slow, nasal, diaphragmatic breathing can reduce sympathetic stress, activate your vagus nerve, and reset your nervous system in minutes.[5]

Just a few rounds of slow, nasal, diaphragmatic breathing can begin to shift your nervous system from bracing to receptive. From frozen to fluid. From survival to stability.

This is why breath isn't just stress management, it's movement preparation. It's the first signal that tells your body: *We're safe now. Let's go.* This aspect of vitality is so important that I have dedicated an entire section of postural alignment rehab, teaching people like you how to breathe intentionally. It has helped people all over the United States to calm their nervous system and help rewire for vitality. I put the full Breath Trio in part 3 of this book, but here's a quick primer.

The Alignment Breath Trio

These aren't hacks, they're tools. Each one targets a different nervous system state and helps your body shift gears the way it was designed to.

- **Navy SEAL Breath** *Regulates the sympathetic nervous system*
  Sharpens focus and builds composure to prepare for added stress or pressure situations. It's a great Monday morning routine. Inhale for four seconds, hold for four, exhale for four, hold again. Repeat three to five times. Simple and powerful.
- **Amen Breath** *Activates the parasympathetic nervous system through the vagus nerve*
  Reset for peace and recovery. Inhale through your nose, exhale slowly with a deep, low "Ahhh-men." Feel the vibration drop you into calm. It activates your vagus nerve and resets your heart rhythm. Also, great for prayer and a state of gratitude/ appreciation.
- **Barrel Breath** *Rebuilds diaphragmatic control and balances autonomic input*
  Restores diaphragmatic power and postural control. Inhale as if expanding a barrel on all sides: front, sides, and back. Exhale

slowly and steadily. This breath does more than calm you; it rebuilds you.

For now, pick one of them and take thirty seconds to breathe with intention. You may be shocked at how infrequently you are engaging your deep muscles of respiration.

Fit While You Sit: Your Micro-Routine Reset

You may not be able to change your job, but you can break the pattern. I used to go into businesses and teach people how to engage their core and stay active, even when tied to a desk for hours on end. Business owners loved it because of the noticeable difference in energy and productivity when employees would actually implement the routine.

If you sit for long periods of time throughout the day, try this every hour:

1. **Boxer's Bounce**—Stand up and assume an athletic position. Bounce back and forth on your toes for ten seconds, like a boxer in the ring. It might feel silly, but it increases lymphatic flow, improves circulation, prevents blood clots, and stimulates cerebrospinal fluid to the brain. Not bad for ten seconds.
2. **Neck circles**—slow, full circles, three in each direction.
3. **Wobble**—use an inflatable disc and go through the wobble routine at www.fxalign.com/wobble
4. **Diaphragmatic breath**—Choose one of the alignment breath trio exercises and take three slow, intentional breaths.

This whole routine takes under two minutes. It resets your posture, wakes up your nervous system, and keeps your body from slipping into shutdown.

And let's be honest, seeing your coworkers doing the boxer's bounce every hour is the kind of weird that makes work fun again. That's a culture builder!

Final Word: Walk Your Way Back to Vitality

You don't need permission to move. You don't need a trainer, an app, or the "right" routine. You need a commitment to show up, breathe, and move like your life depends on it. Because it does.

And once you do, the next piece falls into place: food. When you combine the right movement with the proper fuel, you shift from survival to restoration. But just like movement, food can fuel healing or it can fuel the interference. In the next chapter, we'll show you how to feed your body the way it was designed to be fueled.

CHAPTER 10

Food by God or Food by Man

Our ancestors hunted food. We now hunt for ingredients we can pronounce.
—Unknown

What if I told you the food industry isn't just selling you junk? It's rewriting your biology every time you say yes to it.

Your cravings have become engineered, your hunger has been manipulated, and your metabolism has been hijacked by an industry that puts profits over the welfare of its consumers.[1] All of this has kept you sick, inflamed, and dependent on Medicine.

Here's the truth: Food isn't just fuel, it's a message. Every bite carries biological instructions that interact with your DNA, flipping genetic switches on or off, shaping your energy, brain function, and metabolism at the cellular level.[2] Most people are simply eating the wrong message, feeding their body garbage code. They think they're making healthy choices because they follow social media health trends, read labels, and trust the marketing on their food. But real health doesn't come from a package, it comes from nature.

We've been conditioned to believe food is complicated. Every year, there's a new diet, a new "superfood," a new set of rules. High-carb, low-carb. Plant-based, paleo. But what if it's not that complicated? What if, instead of trying to decode every new health trend, we simplified it down to one essential truth:

There is Food by God, and there is Food by Man.

What Is Food by God?

Food by God is food in its original, natural state, the way it was created and intended to be consumed. It is:

- **Grown in the earth.** Vegetables, fruits, nuts, seeds, and herbs, grown in rich, regenerative soil.
- **Raised naturally.** Grass-fed beef, pastured poultry, wild-caught fish, and raw dairy, animals raised as they were designed to live.
- **Unprocessed and unmanipulated.** No synthetic additives, no artificial preservatives, no food dyes, no chemical-laden substitutions.
- **Fermented and cultured foods.** Traditional lacto-fermented foods such as sauerkraut, kimchi, kefir, and yogurt are rich in enzymes, probiotics, and bioavailable nutrients that support digestion, immunity, and metabolic health.

It is food that nourishes. Food that provides essential nutrients, feeds the microbiome, supports the nervous system, and fuels the body's natural ability to heal.[3] It's not a diet; it's how humans were meant to eat.

What Is Food by Man?

Now, contrast that with Food by Man: food that is man-made, man-ipulated, and man-ufactured for mass consumption and a long shelf life. This includes:

Highly processed foods. Cereals, snack bars, protein shakes, and packaged meals filled with refined sugars and seed oils.
Lab-created ingredients. Artificial sweeteners, chemically extracted vegetable oils, synthetic vitamins, and genetically modi-fied organisms.
Factory-farmed meats. Animals raised in confined spaces, pumped full of antibiotics and hormones, fed an unnatural diet of corn and soy.

Food by Man is everywhere. It's what fills the middle aisles of the grocery store, dominates advertisements, and what most of the population eats daily without question. But here's the kicker: It is engineered for addiction, not for health.[4]

It's not just unhealthy. It's designed to make you crave more, eat more, and stay stuck in metabolic dysfunction. Processed foods are overwhelmingly carb-heavy, spiking insulin and locking you into a cycle of blood sugar crashes and cravings.[5] At the same time, their nutrient density is so low that the opportunity cost of filling your belly with them is devastating to your health.[6] These foods manipulate dopamine, hijacking the brain's reward system in the same way drugs do.[7] Food by Man doesn't just fill shelves. It fills hospitals.

Sayer Ji, founder of GreenMedInfo, puts it this way: "Food contains methyl groups capable of epigenetic modulation of DNA expression."[8] Translation? The food you eat can literally rewrite your genetic future. Every meal is sending signals, either reinforcing health or driving disease. This is why Food by God (whole, unprocessed, nutrient-dense) is vastly different from Food by Man (engineered, synthetic, and stripped of real nutrition). One provides the right biological instructions. The other provides corrupt data, leading to metabolic dysfunction, inflammation, and chronic disease.

And here's where it gets even deeper: exosomes. These tiny, naturally occurring messengers in food don't just deliver nutrients; they carry genetic information that survives digestion and directly influences your cells.[9]

Think of it like a software update.

- Eat the right foods, and you upgrade your system. Your body gets new instructions to repair, regenerate, and thrive. The information signals that the world is at peace and the materials introduced to your microbiome have a symbiotic relationship.
- Eat processed junk, and you download a virus. Your body receives faulty instructions, leading to inflammation, metabolic dysfunction, and disease. The information signals to your existing microbiome that the world is at war and creates unrest from within.

One study even found that exosomal microRNAs from rice can change how the liver controls cholesterol by affecting a specific receptor, the LDL receptor.[10] That means the food you eat isn't just affecting digestion; it's sending signals that alter gene expression by telling your cells to turn certain genes on or off. In other words, the food you eat isn't just affecting your stomach; it's influencing how your body works down to the most intricate level, how you adapt and respond, almost like reprogramming a computer.

Think about that next time you reach for something with an ingredient list longer than your grocery receipt. You're not just eating; you're programming your body. The question is: Are you writing a script to reclaim vitality, or setting yourself up for unnecessary suffering, less energy, and decreased healthy longevity?

Shift Back to Real Food

For most of human history, food was simple. It came straight from the earth, unaltered and nutrient-dense. But then we industrialized it, stripping its nutritional power, loading it with preservatives, and engineering it for convenience rather than health. Now, we live in a world where people are overfed and undernourished, sick but still eating.

Joel Salatin, a pioneer in regenerative farming, puts it bluntly: "Know your food, know your farmer, and know your kitchen."

But most people don't. They've outsourced their food supply to manufacturers, fast-food chains, and factory farmers at best, that prioritize production and profit over nutrients and vitality. They eat what's cheap and convenient, never questioning the long-term effects of factory-made food. They trust labels, but those labels lie, calling processed, chemical-laden foods "heart-healthy" and "natural" when they are anything but. After several generations of being overwhelmed with convenience food, consumers are slowly recognizing that it takes the industry way too long to protect us from known harms, if ever! People caught on to the overuse of antibiotics in our food supply being a detriment to our health, but what is next and how long will it take for knowledge and labeling to catch up? There are fail-safe standards for our own dinner plates that can save us from a lot of diversions in our own health.

The Devastation of Modern Farming

A groundbreaking University of Washington study revealed something alarming: crops grown in regenerative, organic soil contain significantly higher levels of essential nutrients, including magnesium, calcium, potassium, and key vitamins, than conventionally grown food. Meanwhile, industrially farmed crops are depleted, lacking the minerals and antioxidants necessary to fuel the body. Worse, they often contain elevated levels of toxic metals like cadmium and nickel.[11] Unfortunately, these aren't just academic or scientific facts. Mineral deficiencies set you up for many of the biggest battles that we face today including mental health issues, accelerated aging, and disease processes like cancer and chronic fatigue.

Jordan Rubin, founder of Beyond Organic, puts it this way: "You will never be healthier than the soil your food is grown in."[12] The land is sick, and so are we. The explosion of chronic diseases, including diabetes, heart disease, and autoimmune disorders, isn't a mystery. It's the direct result of consuming food that lacks the raw materials needed for vitality.

Salatin drives the point home: "The best way to control your future is to control your food." But most people don't take control because they either don't have the basic knowledge to do so or they are inundated with conflicting guidance. So instead, they eat what's marketed to them: cheap, processed, artificially preserved food products designed for shelf life, not human life.

The Wisdom of Traditional Foods: What We Forgot (and Must Remember)

For generations, humans thrived on diets rich in whole, unprocessed, nutrient-dense foods. Traditional cultures instinctively knew what modern science is rediscovering: real food is the foundation of health, longevity, and vitality. But something happened in the last century. Industrial food production replaced wisdom with convenience, and in the process, we lost something critical: the knowledge of how to nourish ourselves.

Sally Fallon Morell, author of *Nourishing Traditions* and founder of the Weston A. Price Foundation, has spent decades uncovering and reviving the lost dietary wisdom of our ancestors. Drawing from the research of Dr. Weston A. Price, she highlights how indigenous people who consumed their native, whole-food diets had perfect teeth, strong bones, and a complete absence of chronic disease.[13] These populations lived without cavities, degenerative illness, or the metabolic chaos we see today not because they had better genetics, but because they ate foods in their most nourishing, bioavailable forms.

In every traditional culture Dr. Price studied, people prioritized foods rich in fat-soluble vitamins (A, D, E, and K), minerals, and high-quality fats. They consumed:

- Raw, unprocessed dairy: fresh milk, butter, and cheese from pasture-raised animals, loaded with essential fats and probiotics
- Grass-fed and organ meats: liver, bone marrow, and other nutrient-dense cuts, providing a wealth of vitamins and minerals
- Fermented foods: raw sauerkraut, kimchi, kefir, and yogurt, all supporting gut health and digestion
- Soaked and sprouted grains: traditional cultures took extra steps to prepare grains, nuts, and seeds to remove anti-nutrients and make them more digestible
- Bone broths and collagen-rich foods: packed with gelatin, glycine, and amino acids essential for joint health, skin, and digestion

Compare that to today's diet, filled with heavily processed seed oils, refined sugar, and artificial additives, all of which disrupt metabolism, gut health, and neurological function.

The Death of Real Fat: How We Got Duped

Perhaps one of the greatest nutritional tragedies of modern times has been the demonization of healthy fats. Traditional cultures thrived on butter, lard, coconut oil, and animal fats, yet in the twentieth century we were told to fear these foods. Enter margarine, hydrogenated vegetable oils, and chemically altered fats, which fueled a rise in inflammation, heart disease, and metabolic dysfunction.[14]

Sally has been a leading voice in setting the record straight: fats from pastured animals, grass-fed butter, and tropical oils are not the enemy; they are essential for brain function, hormone production, and cellular health. In fact, the fat-soluble vitamins found in these foods (particularly vitamins A, D, and K$_2$) are necessary for the absorption of minerals like calcium and magnesium, which protect against osteoporosis and dental decay. Without these fats, the body cannot properly utilize critical nutrients.

Meanwhile, industrial seed oils such as canola, soybean, and corn oil have quietly poisoned the food supply.[15] These highly processed, oxidized fats disrupt cell membranes, contribute to chronic inflammation, and have been linked to everything from heart disease to autoimmune disorders. Yet they remain a staple in nearly every processed food.

The Resurgence of Traditional Nutrition

The good news? People are waking up. The rise of regenerative farming, raw milk co-ops, and traditional food preparation methods shows that we are rediscovering what our ancestors never forgot: real food heals.

If we want to reclaim vitality, we must reject the industrialized, ultra-processed food system and return to the time-tested principles of traditional diets. That means:

- Choosing grass-fed, pastured meats over factory-farmed protein
- Ditching heavily processed seed oils in favor of animal fats, butter, and coconut oil
- Prioritizing fermented foods to restore gut health
- Seeking raw, unprocessed dairy from healthy animals
- Preparing grains, nuts, and seeds the ancestral way: soak, sprout, or ferment to reduce anti-nutrients

Sally Fallon Morell and the Weston A. Price Foundation have fought tirelessly to bring these truths back into public awareness. We don't need a new diet trend. We don't need another food pyramid designed by processed food lobbyists. We need to return to the way food was meant to be eaten: whole, unprocessed, and deeply nourishing.

The choice is clear: We can keep trusting industrial food companies and government-backed nutrition guidelines that have led to a crisis of chronic disease, or we can look back to the wisdom of traditional cultures:

people who ate real food, lived in vibrant health, and passed down knowledge our modern world has ignored for too long.

The future of health doesn't lie in another lab-created food replacement. It lies in rediscovering the food that has sustained humankind for centuries. It's time to return to what works.

Fasting: The Original Design for Healing

Before there were diet trends, before there was a food pyramid, there was fasting. Built into our biology from the beginning, fasting isn't starvation; it's strategy. It's the body's original blueprint for healing, restoration, and regeneration.

Our ancestors didn't graze all day or snack every two hours. They ate when food was available and fasted when it wasn't. Their bodies adapted, not just to survive, but to thrive during these fasting periods. Today, we have to *choose* what was once automatic: space between meals, time for the body to repair, and the metabolic switch that flips when food is withheld.

That's exactly what fasting does today: it forces your body to flip the metabolic switch from sugar-burning to fat-burning. That's when ketosis kicks in: your body starts running on ketones instead of glucose, unlocking a cleaner, more efficient energy source.[16] But fasting isn't just about weight loss.

Autophagy: Your Body's Built-In Detox and Repair System

A *Nature Cell Biology* study confirmed that fasting triggers a process called autophagy. Autophagy is your body's self-cleaning mode: it breaks down damaged cells, eliminates toxins, and regenerates healthier ones.[17] It's how your body fights off disease, slows aging, and rebuilds itself from the inside out. The result? More energy, less inflammation, and better metabolic health.

If you want to age slower, think clearer, and avoid degenerative disease, autophagy is your best friend. And fasting is how you turn it on. The catch? You can't activate autophagy if you're always eating. Every time you snack, every time you hit that late-night craving, you shut down your body's chance to fully heal. Fasting forces the body to repair instead of just digesting.

What happens if you never fast? Your body never gets the chance to clean house. The damage builds up. Cells malfunction, inflammation sets in, and your nervous system no longer feels safe. Fasting isn't deprivation, it's giving your body a chance to take out the trash and feel at ease again. There isn't just one way to fast. The key is to find a rhythm that works for you.

The Different Ways to Fast

- *Intermittent Fasting (IF):* The easiest way to start fasting. You eat within a six- to eight-hour window and fast the rest of the time (typically 16:8 or 18:6). This approach:
  - Activates ketosis
  - Improves insulin sensitivity
  - Supports fat loss without slowing digestion
- *One Meal a Day (OMAD):* OMAD takes intermittent fasting to the next level. You eat one massive, nutrient-dense meal a day and fast for twenty-three hours. Benefits?
  - Deeper ketosis
  - Maximum autophagy activation
  - Mental clarity and laser focus
- *Extended Fasting:* Going beyond twenty-four to seventy-two hours shifts the body into full repair mode. Research shows extended fasting:
  - Destroys precancerous cells
  - Rebuilds the immune system
  - Regenerates damaged tissues

Longer fasts should be done strategically: This isn't about starvation to lose weight; it's about hacking your body's repair system for deep healing.

Why Women Need a Different Approach to Fasting

Women's hormones don't respond to fasting the same way men's do. Women should be strategic about when and how they fast. Dr. Mindy Pelz, a fasting expert and author of *Fast Like a Girl*, explains that fasting affects progesterone, estrogen, and cortisol, and fasting at the wrong time of the month can backfire.[18]

Fasting is a powerful tool for women, but it must be done strategically to work with, not against, hormonal cycles. Dr. Mindy has done an incredible job breaking this down in *Fast Like a Girl*, offering a deep dive into the science of fasting for women, when to push, when to pull back, and how to sync fasting with the menstrual cycle for maximum benefits. This section gives you a high-level overview, but if you want to truly master fasting as a woman, her book is the ultimate guide.

The best times for women to fast longer than fifteen hours:

- Menstruation and early follicular phase (days 1–10)
- Luteal phase, before premenstrual period (days 16–19)

Ignoring these cycles can wreck metabolism, increase stress hormones, and tank energy. Fasting is a weapon, but you have to use it wisely. If your cycles are irregular or absent, that's a sign your body is already under stress; fasting too aggressively can make it worse. Focus on shorter fasts, nourishing foods, and restoring balance before moving into longer windows.

Fasting for Men: The Testosterone Factor

Men can fast more aggressively, but here's the mistake guys make: fasting too much and refueling with Food by Man or carbohydrates. If you refuel incorrectly, you can crash testosterone and wreck muscle mass.

- Intermittent fasting? Great.
- OMAD a few times a week or an occasional extended fast? Solid.
- Extended Fasts followed by Food by Man? Horrible.

Men need to fast, but feast strategically. Load up on pastured meats, wild-caught fish, and healthy fats during eating windows to keep testosterone strong. Fasting is about resilience, not running on fumes. (I'm talking to you, Mr. "All or Nothing.")

But here's the most important thing: listen to your body. Fasting is a tool, not a punishment. Done right, it will transform your metabolism, sharpen your brain, and unlock your body's built-in healing.

Fat-First Fueling: The Healing Strategy after Fasting

After fasting, your body is primed for restoration. This is where food matters most. You don't refuel with junk, you build with intention. We call this approach Fat-First Fueling.

The body was designed to burn fat as a clean, stable fuel source. When you begin your eating window with healthy fats like pastured meats, wild-caught fish, avocado, grass-fed butter, and coconut oil, you generate ketones. These aren't just energy molecules; they're signaling molecules that activate healing across multiple systems. Ketones reduce inflammation, stabilize brain chemistry, and trigger the release of brain-derived neurotrophic factor (BDNF), which supports cognitive repair and resilience.

Even more remarkable, ketosis activates stem cell regeneration. Extended fasts with fat-first fueling renew the body, replacing damaged cells with new ones. This isn't just disease prevention; it's deep healing at the cellular level.

This isn't keto the way Instagram sells it, with bacon wraps or processed cream cheese bombs. Fat-first fueling is simply eating according to the primal design, starting with food that restores. It prioritizes nutrient-dense, unprocessed foods that emphasize fat as the dominant energy source while strategically cycling in nutrient-rich carbohydrates. Seasonal fruits, tubers, and fermented grains have their place, especially for thyroid and hormonal support but fat is the base, not the afterthought.

Traditional cultures did this instinctively. They consumed wild meats, fermented vegetables, seasonal roots, and full-fat dairy, foods rich in fat-soluble vitamins, trace minerals, and metabolic cofactors. This kind of nourishment supports hormone production, brain health, and mitochondrial repair. It works because it honors how the body was designed to fuel and heal.

Ketones and the Brain: Why Your Mind Thrives on Fat

The brain doesn't just tolerate ketones, it prefers them. A 2025 study on bipolar disorder found that a ketogenic state significantly improved both mental and physical health, stabilizing mood where medications often fall short.[19] Other studies show similar improvements for anxiety, depression, schizophrenia, and even Alzheimer's.[20]

A 2024 Stanford study confirmed what vitalistic-minded people have known for decades: shifting the body into ketosis improves brain metabolism and reduces mental illness severity.[21] A *Nature* study found nearly 50 percent of epileptic patients experienced a dramatic drop in seizures on a ketogenic diet, with many seeing over 90 percent reduction.[22] That's not theory. That's hard data.

We've been told psychiatric issues are chemical imbalances requiring lifelong medication. But what if the problem isn't just the brain, it's the fuel that the brain is using for energy?

When we eat Food by God (pastured meats, wild fish, and real fats), we stabilize neurotransmitters, protect the brain, and lower inflammation. When we eat Food by Man (processed sugar, seed oils, and synthetic additives), we create metabolic and nervous system chaos. Ketones bring order to the brain. They're the brain's natural stabilizer.

Fueling for Insulin Sensitivity and Hormonal Repair

Fat-first fueling isn't just about the brain, though. It's one of the most effective strategies for reversing insulin resistance and Type 2 diabetes. A 2022 study in *Frontiers in Psychiatry* found that a ketogenic approach not only improved blood sugar regulation but also reduced depression in diabetic patients.[23] Over half no longer met the criteria for depression after just ten weeks.

A 2021 study in *Signal Transduction and Targeted Therapy* showed that ketosis dramatically improves glucose control by reducing blood sugar and lowering the insulin-to-glucagon ratio.[24] That's the ratio that controls fat burning.

But this only works if your fuel is clean. Dirty keto (processed meats, factory cheese, artificial sweeteners) creates new problems. Fat-first fueling means food by God: real, whole, and healing.

This is about breaking free. Your body already knows how to heal itself. You just have to stop getting in the way. Eat real food. Fast strategically. Let your body do what it was designed to do.

That's how you take control of your health, on your terms.

Transforming Your Relationship with Food

Now it's time to take action, not by overhauling everything overnight, but by becoming aware of how food is shaping your health. Before you dive into strict meal plans or fasting schedules, you need to understand where your food is coming from, what's actually in it, and how your eating patterns are affecting your body. This isn't just about what you eat, it's about how you eat.

In part 3, I'll give you a step-by-step challenge and a full food plan to take this to the next level. But don't jump ahead. If you skip to the "rules" without the right mindset, you'll treat this like another diet instead of the metabolic reset it's meant to be. Right now, your job is to pay attention and start shifting how you think about food.

Here's how to get started:

Step 1: Track Every Bite. Write down everything you eat and where it came from. Factory? Farm? Lab? If you don't know, find out. This isn't forever but it is a good practice for four to six weeks to hold yourself accountable for *knowing* what you eat and truly choosing what enters and integrates with your body.

Check your pantry, fridge, and what's on your plate. If you don't recognize an ingredient, your body won't either. Start shifting toward Food by God: real, unprocessed, nutrient-dense foods that nourish, not deplete.

Step 2: Read Every Label. If it has more than five ingredients, question it. If you can't pronounce something, ditch it.

This habit alone will radically change what you put in your body. The food industry hides garbage under fancy branding and marketing. Don't fall for it. You deserve better.

Step 3: Push yourself into fasting. Skip snacks. Delay breakfast. Try a 16:8 fasting window to feasting window. Remember your fast starts when you stop eating for the day and continues through your sleep.

Fasting isn't about starving yourself, it's about retraining your body to burn fat for fuel and breaking free from the modern addiction to constant eating. Start small and build from there.

BONUS CHALLENGE: Try a Food by God OMAD Monday: one nutrient-dense meal, packed with life-giving foods to fuel, restore, and energize. This isn't about punishment or deprivation. This is one of the sharpest tools you have to break free from unhealthy cravings and metabolic imbalances and reclaim your health. Your body already knows how to heal itself if you will get out of the way.

What you eat can either heal or harm, but it's not the only daily input shaping your biology. Pesticides in your produce are a risk factor. We cannot rely on the things on the shelves to be safe by default. The regulatory agencies need dramatic reform, and our vigilance is necessary when it comes to avoidable but hidden toxic exposure. From the fluoride in your water to the phthalates in your shampoo to the nonstick coating on your pans and the chemicals in your cleaning supplies, the average American is bombarded every day with synthetic compounds that tax your detox pathways. In the next chapter, we'll expose the most common environmental toxins, where they hide, how they affect your health, and the simple steps you can take to reduce your load and reclaim vitality.

CHAPTER 11

Toxic Overload: Why Your Environment Is Making You Sick

Take care of your body, it's the only place you have to live.
—Jim Rohne

We live in a world where chronic disease is the norm. Most people accept that diagnosis is just a matter of time. But very few are asking *why* the body breaks down in the first place.

This chapter is not about spiraling into fear. It's about taking control. It's about recognizing and reducing the toxic burdens that interfere with your body's God-given ability to adapt, detox, and heal. Because here's the reality: we are swimming in toxic soup.

A Toxic World

Since World War II, more than 70,000 chemicals have been introduced into commercial use in the United States. More than 10,000 are used in food processing and packaging alone. According to the EPA, indoor air can be up to one hundred times more toxic than outdoor air.[1] And nearly every home in America is filled with chemical-laden products, from cleaning sprays to cosmetics, cookware to colognes.

But your body isn't numb to these toxins the way our culture is. Your body is screaming, waving red flags. And eventually, it breaks down under the weight of it.

The Danger of Bioaccumulation

One of the most dangerous features of modern toxicity is bioaccumulation: the gradual buildup of toxic substances in the body over time. Unlike acute poisoning, which is immediate and obvious, bioaccumulation happens silently. Toxins are absorbed faster than they are eliminated, leading to a toxic load that increases with age and ongoing exposure. This is particularly dangerous with fat-soluble toxins like dioxins, PCBs, heavy metals, and certain pesticides that lodge in fatty tissues, including the brain and reproductive organs.

A CDC biomonitoring report found detectable levels of over 400 synthetic chemicals in Americans, including flame retardants, phthalates, and perfluorinated chemicals (PFCs), many of which are known to be carcinogenic, neurotoxic, or endocrine-disrupting.[2] In another study, Environmental Working Group found an average of over two hundred industrial chemicals, pollutants, and pesticides in newborn umbilical cord blood, showing that babies are being born pre-polluted.[3]

A 2023 review published in *Environmental Research* linked long-term exposure to persistent organic pollutants (POPs) with increased risk of Type 2 diabetes, metabolic dysfunction, and neurodegenerative disease, even decades after initial exposure.[4]

These chemicals accumulate not only in our bodies but also in the food chain, leading to intergenerational toxicity. What our great-grandmothers were never exposed to, our children are born carrying. This is why reducing exposure (especially in the home!) is so essential. It's not just about feeling better today. It's about protecting the future.

Brain Disease, Cancer, and Common Toxins

Mounting scientific evidence connects everyday environmental toxins to neurodegenerative diseases and cancer. A groundbreaking study published in the *Journal of Alzheimer's Disease* found a "close association" between human exposure to aluminum and familial Alzheimer's, with researchers identifying "significant accumulations" of aluminum in brain tissue from multiple family members who died with the disease.[5]

Notably, aluminum is a common adjuvant in vaccines, including annual flu shots, which are administered widely to children and seniors despite growing concerns about cumulative exposure and brain health. The blood-brain barrier, meant to protect against such intrusions, becomes more permeable with age and inflammation, compounding risk.

Meanwhile, the connection between environmental toxins and cancer continues to be substantiated by robust reviews. Cochrane researchers, known for their rigorous, independent analysis, have identified strong evidence linking certain chemicals like benzene (a known carcinogen found in air pollution and household cleaners) and formaldehyde (common in building materials and personal care products) to elevated cancer risk.[6] In their review of pesticide exposure, the Cochrane Database highlighted significantly higher risks of leukemia and non-Hodgkin's lymphoma in individuals regularly exposed to herbicides and insecticides, particularly in agricultural and landscaping professions.[7]

These findings reinforce a clear message: exposure to common environmental toxins isn't benign. It's bioactive, cumulative, and in many cases, carcinogenic or neurotoxic. Choosing cleaner products and minimizing exposure isn't fear-based; it's evidence-based stewardship of our physical bodies and minds.

Your Detox System

The great news is that your body is a detox machine. Nine major organs are involved in the detoxification process:

- Liver: Your master detoxifier. It processes everything (food, air, chemicals) and removes waste through bile and feces.
- Kidneys: Filter two hundred quarts of blood daily, eliminating waste through urine.
- Lungs: Filter toxins from the air and blood.
- Lymphatic System: Gathers toxins and sends them to the liver.
- Blood-Brain Barrier: Shields the brain from chemical intrusion.
- Gallbladder: Works with the liver to remove waste via bile.

- Fat Cells: Store toxins to keep them from damaging vital organs.
- Intestines: Eliminate waste and play a major role in detox.
- Skin: Absorbs and excretes toxins.

But this system works best when it isn't overwhelmed. Most Americans consume foods devoid of quality nutrients and are chronically exposed to chemicals. Without the raw materials (like zinc, selenium, vitamin C, and amino acids), your body can't detox effectively. When there's more coming in than the body can get out, toxicity sets in.

The Role of Oxidative Stress

When toxins flood the body faster than it can remove them, free radicals increase, and antioxidants can't keep up. This leads to *oxidative stress*, a state of chronic low-grade cellular damage that accelerates aging and fuels disease.

Normally, your body produces free radicals through everyday processes like metabolism and exercise, and it neutralizes them with antioxidants from nutrients like vitamin C, vitamin E, selenium, and plant polyphenols. But when toxins flood in and nutrients are depleted, antioxidants can't keep up.

Oxidative stress disrupts nearly every system:

- It damages DNA
- Impairs mitochondrial function
- Inhibits detox pathways
- Triggers inflammation

It's a silent drain on your vitality, but it's *almost* completely preventable.

The Unavoidable Burden

You can't avoid every toxin. Air pollution from cars, airplanes, factories, building materials, and even natural exposures like radon and mold circulate through our atmosphere daily. Increasingly, our air is also being impacted by the aerosolization of heavy metals and other chemicals through geoengineering and weather manipulation practices, adding to the burden of airborne toxins we inhale. Water pollution from pesticides, industrial runoff, prescription medications in sewage, chlorine, fluoride, and heavy metals can enter our bodies through drinking, bathing, and cooking. These pollutants often make their way into the soil, eventually contaminating our food supply.

At the same time, we are constantly bathed in electromagnetic radiation from cell phones, Wi-Fi routers, smart devices, and 5G infrastructure, with growing concerns about long-term effects on cellular function and oxidative stress. Many of these exposures generate free radicals in the body, contributing to chronic inflammation, cellular damage, and disease.

Symptoms of Toxic Load

If you have experienced any of the following in the last six months, you might be suffering from overexposure to toxins. And if you identify with two or more, your toxic load may be impacting your body's ability to thrive:

- Fatigue or low energy
- Hormone imbalance
- Brain fog
- Sleep disruption
- Digestive issues
- Skin problems
- Trouble losing weight
- Anxiety or mood swings

Toxicity isn't just physical. It affects mood, cognition, hormones, and energy in ways you never imagined possible.

The Hormone Disruption Crisis

Toxins interfere with your body's internal communication system, especially your hormones. And hormonal problems are now rampant. The evidence is everywhere.

- Polycystic ovary syndrome (PCOS)

- Early puberty
- Endometriosis
- Infertility
- Low Testosterone (in both men and women)
- Declining sperm counts and reduced motility
- Rising testicular dysfunction

This isn't alarmism. It's measurable.

Studies show a staggering 50–60 percent decline in sperm count across Western countries in recent decades.[8] Multiple human IVF cohorts show higher exposure to phthalates and BPA is associated with lower fertility and live birth rates.[9] When chemical exposures begin in utero, as confirmed in the intersex birth study, the disrupted development not only sets a lifelong course for reproductive dysfunction but also highlights why these conditions often feel systemic, not isolated.[10]

A Generational Tipping Point

A common critique we hear is, *"Grandma used bleach, ate margarine, and lived into her nineties."*

But Grandma wasn't born with pesticides in her bloodstream. She didn't grow up eating ultra-processed food. Her body didn't endure the daily barrage of chemicals from modern packaging, plastics, air pollution, and wireless radiation.

Toxicity builds across decades and across generations. This isn't about longevity. It's about *healthy longevity.* And by that measure, Americans rank dead last among high-income countries, spending an average of 12.4 years in bad health, managing disease at the end of life.

Final Shift: From Tolerating to Targeting

You were not designed to simply manage disease. You were designed to express vitality. But to do that, you have to stop tolerating what's common. You have to stop normalizing chronic symptoms. And you have to stop outsourcing your health to a system that rarely addresses root causes.

It's not enough to eat well and exercise. You need to *remove interference.*

Next: Your Home Detox

In the next chapter, we'll walk through the seven most common environmental exposures hiding in plain sight, and show you exactly how to replace them with cleaner, safer, vitality-supporting alternatives.

This isn't about achieving perfection. It's about reducing the unnecessary load your body carries every single day. Let's start there.

CHAPTER 12

The Home Detox: Practical Swaps to Clean Up Your Environment

Reducing exposure to environmental toxins in the home is one of the simplest and most effective steps we can take for long-term health.
—Dr. Andrew Weil

You can't control everything you're exposed to. But what happens inside your home? That's within your reach.

This chapter gives you the seven most impactful places to reduce your toxic burden. The goal isn't to become a purist. It's to stop sabotaging your biology with products and exposures that were never meant to be part of human life. You can do this without fear, without perfectionism, and without overwhelm.

If you've ever asked, "Where do I even start?" this is where. You might have started long ago, but still asking, "What might I be missing?" This chapter will expose hidden offenders.

Minimizing Toxins Happens Largely at Home

We sleep on mattresses treated with flame-retardant chemicals, wake up groggy because those same toxins disrupt thyroid function, and reach for water bottled in plastic that leaches phthalates. Our morning routine layers on more: fluoride and chlorine in tap water, mouthwash and toothpaste spiked with artificial colors and sweeteners, deodorants packed with aluminum and parabens, and lotions that drive these chemicals deeper into the skin. The average American uses nine personal care products per day, containing about 126 toxic ingredients.[1]

By the time we're dressed in synthetic fabrics or dry-cleaned clothes, we've already absorbed dozens of possible carcinogens, hormone disruptors, and neurotoxins. Add in a quick breakfast of processed cereal, lunch meat, or diet soda (laden with pesticides, additives, and artificial sweeteners), and the burden climbs higher.

All this before most people even leave the house.

The good news is that your body is designed to filter and handle a certain toxic load. Our goal isn't to eliminate every toxin in our environment. It's to minimize exposure by eliminating the ones we are aware of. What you eat and drink is a great starting point.

#1. What You Eat and Drink

Food-related toxins aren't just in the food, they are added to food, in food packaging, used to preserve food and to grow food. These additives are designed to manipulate flavor, preserve shelf life, and make processed food more addictive. The list is too long to absorb but some of the top offenders to be aware of that will help you avoid the wrong foods all together and significantly reduce your toxic burden in your diet are:

- Monosodium glutamate (MSG)
- Aspartame and other artificial sweeteners like sucralose and saccharin
- Nitrates
- Synthetic colors
- Hydrogenated or partially hydrogenated oils (trans fats)
- High-fructose corn syrup
- Seed oils (canola, soybean, corn, cottonseed, etc.)
- Preservatives like BHA, BHT, sodium benzoate
- Genetically modified foods

Identifying and avoiding these chemicals is not always as easy as it should be. MSG, for example, is classified as an excitotoxin,[2] meaning it overstimulates brain cells (especially in children!) and can trigger symptoms like headaches, brain fog, anxiety, fatigue, and mood swings. Here's the catch, even if a product does not have "MSG," it might still contain it, just disguised under another one of the long list of names for MSG: hydrolyzed vegetable protein, autolyzed yeast, yeast extract, soy protein isolate, calcium caseinate, "natural flavor," glutamic acid, textured protein, disodium guanylate, or disodium inosinate.

The best option, however, is to shift away from processed foods and to real foods. Then skip conventional produce and agriculture because not all produce and animal products are equal depending on farming practices. The same chemicals used to combat weeds, pests, rot, and fungus are endocrine-disrupting chemicals (EDCs), which hijack your nervous system and cause cancer.

Eating clean doesn't have to be complicated. Look for the USDA Organic seal when buying packaged food, avoid ultra-processed options, and prioritize fresh, whole, real food. Even better, form a relationship with your local farmers and go purchase directly from them.

Pro Tip: Set food boundaries. Know your nonnegotiables. Don't make exceptions just because it's convenient. We don't eat fast food, period. Not because we're better but because it's easier to say no once than to debate every time.

#2. What Goes on Your Skin

What goes on your skin gets in your body. Your skin is your largest organ, and it's not an impermeable barrier, it's a sponge. Just as a nicotine patch or birth control patch is absorbed through the skin, your personal care products are likely making their way into your body and influencing your function.

According to a study by Environmental Defence, 96 percent of makeup products tested contained lead, 90 percent contained beryllium, 61 percent contained thallium, 51 percent contained cadmium, and 20 percent contained arsenic.[3] Daily-use products like shampoo, lotion, deodorant, toothpaste, sunscreen, and makeup are among the most concentrated sources of EDCs in your home.[4] That includes:

- Parabens and phthalates (hormone disruptors)

- Synthetic fragrance/parfum (often 100+ undisclosed chemicals)
- Heavy metals (lead, cadmium, mercury)
- SLS/SLES (skin irritants and chemical carriers)
- Formaldehyde-releasing preservatives
- Petrolatum/mineral oil

Reviewing the labels of personal care products is not as easy as food because chemistry and botanical terms can be confusing and hard to pronounce. Some red flag root words and naming clues in the ingredients include:

- "Fragrance" or "parfum"*
- -paraben
- -pthalate
- Phenol / phenoxy-
- -oxyeth- / -eth (like laureth, ceteareth, polyethylene glycol/PEG)
- -siloxane / -methicone (like cyclopentasiloxane, dimethicone)
- Triclosan / Triclocarban
- Benz- / -benzene / -benzoate
- Talc

Cleaner swaps:
Use EWG's SkinDeep® database or MadeSafe.org to find vetted brands. Transparency matters more than marketing.

*Fragrances: the term fragrance on a label is legally protected as a trade secret, which means companies can hide dozens or even hundreds of undisclosed chemicals under that single term. Many of these are linked to hormone-disrupting chemicals, allergic reactions, headaches, respiratory issues, developmental toxicity, and bioaccumulation.[5] Phthalates are often used to make the scent last longer and these types of chemicals have been found in human breast milk, blood, and even umbilical cord samples highlighting the systemic and bioaccumulative effects. The term fragrance is a huge red flag. The good news is that there are some fragrance products that are free from phthalates, parabens, and synthetic musks.

Artificial fragrances are found in everything from perfumes, deodorants and shampoos to lotions, and sunscreens. Once inside your home, the scents off-gas volatile organic compounds (VOCs), which are pollutants that linger in your air, settle into dust, and are inhaled or absorbed through the skin. VOC exposure has been linked to asthma, headaches, allergic reactions, mood disruption, and developmental harm, especially in children.

Removing artificial fragrance from your home is one of the most effective and immediate ways to reduce your toxic burden. It clears the air, supports hormone health, protects developing children, and restores your body's ability to detect what's clean, safe, and supportive of vitality. Clean doesn't have a smell, clean is the absence of toxicity. Look for products labeled "fragrance-free" or those that disclose every ingredient. Don't be fooled by vague marketing terms like "natural scent," they're often unregulated and misleading.

Deodorant: This is an important choice because it is applied daily to a sensitive area near lymph nodes. Aluminum compounds are present in conventional deodorants, and they clog pores, disrupt hormones, create breast cancer concerns and potential neurotoxicity.[6] For example, triclosan is linked to thyroid dysfunction and antibiotic resistance. Once again, look for full ingredient transparency, no hidden fragrance, aluminum-free, natural ingredients, no parabens, phthalates, triclosan, PEGs, or synthetic dyes.

Toothpaste: conventional toothpaste almost always contains harmful ingredients like fluoride (a known neurotoxin), SLS (a harsh foaming agent), triclosan, artificial sweeteners, and dyes.[7] A clean toothpaste should be fluoride-free, SLS-free, and made with natural minerals like hydroxyapatite, essential oils, and herbal extracts and have full ingredient transparency.

Shampoo: Conventional shampoos are loaded with sulfates, parabens, and synthetic fragrance full of toxins. A clean shampoo should be sulfate-free, fragrance-free, or scented with essential oils, and made with plant-based cleansers and nourishing botanicals. Look for brands that prioritize scalp health and reducing toxic load.

Anything that goes on your body should be assessed in a similar manner to the products above.

#3. Cleaning Products

Walk down any cleaning aisle and you'll be hit with the scent of lemon, lavender, or linen, but behind the pleasant fragrance is often a cocktail of chemicals with no place in a healthy home. Somewhere along the way, we traded common sense for convenience, prioritizing "no germs" and "no grime" over the simple goal of avoiding poison. Yet those same products we use to disinfect countertops and scrub sinks may be harming our bodies far more than the bacteria we're trying to eliminate. Cleaning products are a major, and often overlooked, contributor to toxic load, affecting everything from respiratory function to hormone balance and gut integrity. Many of these substances are volatile organic compounds (VOCs) that release toxic fumes, linger in indoor air, and are absorbed through skin contact or inhalation.[8]

The laundry room is a powerful place to start. Your laundry detergent and dryer sheets are two of the most impactful first swaps you can make to significantly reduce the toxic burden on your body. Conventional detergents and fresh-smelling dryer sheets are often laced with harsh chemicals, including:

- Perchloroethylene (PERC): A neurotoxic dry-cleaning solvent linked to liver and kidney damage and classified as a likely human carcinogen by the EPA.
- Formaldehyde: Common in detergents and air fresheners to preserve fragrance, but it's also a known human carcinogen and respiratory irritant.
- Chlorine: Used in bleach and disinfectants, it can form toxic by-products like chloroform and dioxins that damage the liver and disrupt thyroid function.
- Ammonia: Found in glass cleaners and degreasers, it can trigger asthma attacks and irritate the eyes, skin, and respiratory system.
- Fragrance: *see above in personal care.*

These ingredients are not just skin or lung irritants; they can interfere with hormonal signaling, burden liver detox pathways, and even compromise the gut microbiome, which is critical for immune function, digestion, and brain health. Research shows that exposure to cleaning sprays and disinfectants can damage gut flora and increase the risk for autoimmune conditions, asthma, and metabolic dysfunction, even among otherwise healthy individuals.[9]

Clean swaps:
- White vinegar + water (1:4 ratio) instead of bleach
- Baking soda and castile soap instead of abrasive chemical cleaners
- Essential oils for scent (tea tree, lemon, eucalyptus) instead of fragrances
- Wool dryer balls instead of dryer sheets
- Honest brands: Branch Basics, Norwex, GreenShield

Greenwashing is rampant in the cleaning product industry, so don't rely on pretty packaging of fresh open meadows and flowers or on vague claims of "natural." If the label doesn't list every ingredient, put it back on the shelf.

#4. Cookware and Food Storage
You might be eating organic chicken, but if you're cooking it on a scratched nonstick pan or storing leftovers in plastic, you're still ingesting toxins.

Many common kitchen items, especially those coated in nonstick chemicals or made of plastic, can leach EDCs and potentially carcinogenic substances into the food you eat, especially when exposed to heat. One of the most well-known concerns is Teflon, the nonstick coating made with perfluorooctanoic acid (PFOA), a chemical belonging to the larger class of PFAS, also known as "forever chemicals."[10] In one tragic case from West Virginia, hundreds of people in Parkersburg developed thyroid disease, testicular cancer, and pregnancy complications after years of exposure to PFOA-contaminated water caused by DuPont's Teflon plant.[11] The story became the basis for the 2019 film *Dark Waters* and prompted a series of lawsuits and government crackdowns on PFAS contamination.

Even beyond nonstick coatings, cookware made from aluminum or copper can pose risks if not properly coated, as these metals can leach into food during cooking, especially when acidic ingredients like tomatoes or vinegar are used. A 2017 study published in *Science of The Total Environment* found measurable aluminum migration from cookware into food under regular cooking conditions, contributing to neurotoxicity and oxidative stress.[12] Heating aluminum or touching aluminum to hot food is a boundary we don't cross in our household.

And in the realm of food storage, reheating food in plastic containers, even "microwave-safe" ones, can release phthalates and bisphenols, both of which are known endocrine disruptors linked to reproductive harm and metabolic disorders.[13]

Choosing the right materials is essential for reducing exposure. Cast iron is naturally nonstick once seasoned and adds trace iron to the diet, which is beneficial for most people. Stainless steel is nonreactive, durable, and doesn't leach chemicals into food. Ceramic cookware, when lead-free and properly manufactured, provides an inert surface free of chemical coatings. For storage, glass containers are completely nonreactive, microwave-safe, and long-lasting. Silicone storage bags and lids are flexible and heat-resistant alternatives to plastic, provided they're 100 percent food-grade. These seemingly small swaps have a powerful cumulative effect, and for families trying to reduce their toxic burden, the kitchen is one of the best places to start.

Cookware to avoid:
- Teflon (PFOA/PFAS)
- Aluminum (uncoated)
- Copper (unlined)

Safer choices:
- Cast iron
- Stainless steel
- Lead-free ceramic
- Glass

Storage upgrades:
- Ditch plastic. Use glass containers and silicone lids.
- Avoid reheating anything in plastic or styrofoam.
- Use beeswax wrap instead of plastic wrap.

These are small swaps but provide a big impact, especially when done consistently over time.

#5. Your Home Water Supply

The average American is exposed to an estimated twenty-five gallons of contaminated water every day.[14] That includes drinking, bathing, brushing your teeth, cooking, washing your hands, and doing laundry. Water touches nearly every system in your body, and yet most people never give it a second thought.

Public water systems are legally allowed to contain thousands of contaminants, including:

- Chlorine and chloroform
- Pesticides
- PFAS ("forever chemicals")
- Volatile Organic Compounds (VOCs)
- Heavy metals (lead, arsenic, mercury)
- Pharmaceutical residues (birth control, antidepressants, statins)
- Fluoride

Absorption Is Not Just Oral, It's Also through Skin and Lungs

One of the most overlooked facts about water toxicity is this: you absorb water-based toxins through your skin and lungs.

A fifteen-minute hot shower can be the toxic equivalent of drinking eight full glasses of unfiltered tap water. That's due to both dermal absorption and steam inhalation.[15] One of the worst offenders is chloroform, a known carcinogen that vaporizes during hot water use and can linger in bathrooms long after the water is off.

Children are especially vulnerable. Their smaller body mass and thinner skin make them absorb more relative to weight, and their detox pathways are less developed.

Studies have linked chronic exposure to VOCs and chlorine by-products in water to:

- Hormonal disruption

- Reproductive dysfunction
- Neurological damage
- Immune suppression
- Cancer

Fluoride Is Bad. Dirty Fluoride Is Worse

You've probably heard that fluoride is added to water to prevent cavities. What you probably haven't heard is that the fluoride used in municipal systems isn't pharmaceutical grade, it's a by-product of industrial phosphate fertilizer production, often contaminated with arsenic, lead, and radionuclides. It's not just unnecessary, it's harmful.

Multiple peer-reviewed studies have confirmed that fluoride is a neurotoxin, especially dangerous for developing brains.[16] Prenatal and early childhood exposure is now linked to:

- Lower IQ scores
- Impaired cognitive function
- Neurodevelopmental delays

The National Toxicology Program, a federal body, released a landmark review in 2024 acknowledging this risk.[17] Still, the CDC and EPA have failed to act. We've seen this battle firsthand. At Stand for Health Freedom, we supported local activists in Florida who successfully removed fluoride in over a dozen municipalities. That momentum led to a statewide ban on water fluoridation in 2024, second only to Utah.

Here's the ethical bottom line: **Water should hydrate, not medicate.** You deserve informed consent, not mass medication through your tap.

What You Can Do

Best water sources:
- **Verified spring water** (ideal but not always accessible)
- **Reverse osmosis (RO)** filters (removes 99 percent of toxins, including fluoride, PFAS, lead, and pharmaceuticals)
- **Gravity-fed systems** like Berkey or AquaTru (portable and highly effective)

At minimum, install an under-sink RO system for drinking and cooking water. If budget allows, consider a whole-house system to filter both hot and cold water at the point of entry.

But drinking water is only half the equation.

Your skin absorbs toxins in the shower and bath too.

Next steps:
- Add a shower filter to remove chlorine, fluoride, and sediment
- Install a bathtub faucet filter if your kids soak regularly
- Use EWG's Water Filter Buying Guide or the NSF Certified Product Listings to find filters that meet your needs
- Look up your local water quality at ewg.org/tapwater

#6. Air Quality in Your Home

Indoor air is two to five times more polluted than outdoor air, yet we spend 90 percent of our time indoors. Household dust alone harbors a toxic cocktail: studies routinely detect ten or more harmful chemicals (including flame retardants, phthalates, VOCs, pesticides, lead, mercury, and arsenic) in nearly every US home.[18] Dust isn't just dirt, it becomes an airborne chemical delivery system that accumulates over time, undermining vitality.

Ventilate and Filter: A Two-Pronged Approach

Improving indoor air quality isn't just about removing toxins, it's also about keeping fresh air flowing so that the toxicity level of your air doesn't snowball and remain stagnant. Ventilation, whether by opening windows or using exhaust fans, prevents toxins from accumulating. When fresh air intake isn't possible due to pollution or allergens, HEPA and MERV-rated filters serve as a crucial companion. Portable HEPA cleaners have been shown to significantly reduce indoor particulate levels, improve nasal and respiratory symptoms in susceptible individuals, and significantly reduce asthmatic events in children.[19] Central HVAC systems outfitted with MERV 13 filters can reduce up to 85 percent of fine particles.

Your air quality is improved by commonsense actions too. Vacuuming, dusting, or even moving carpets stirs up dangerous particles in the air, especially if your vacuum lacks a HEPA filter. So it makes sense to run a HEPA air purifier on high settings during cleaning to capture these airborne irritants before they settle or are inhaled.

Greenery with Perspective: Houseplants Support, but Don't Replace

The benefits of houseplants for health and well-being are well-established. Numerous studies show that indoor plants can help regulate humidity, reduce airborne dust, and even lower levels of stress, anxiety, and mental fatigue. Certain plants (i.e., peace lilies, spider plants, and snake plants) contribute to microbial balance by suppressing airborne mold and bacteria. While you'd need hundreds of plants to purify air like a HEPA filter, even a few strategically placed ones can create a calming, life-giving atmosphere that supports mental health and complements a clean indoor environment.

A Blueprint for Clean Indoor Air

Clean indoor air is a cornerstone of maintaining low toxic load and supporting vitality. Aim for a clean-air foundation by:

1. Eliminating artificial fragrances
2. Increasing ventilation
3. Upgrading to HEPA and MERV-13 filtration
4. Running purifiers during cleaning
5. Supplementing with houseplants

Your body is exposed to everything it breathes, so making the air in your home as clean as the food on your table is one of the most effective ways to protect your health, support hormonal balance, and foster long-term well-being.

#7. EMF (Electromagnetic Frequency)

Electromagnetic frequency (EMF) is one of the most overlooked environmental toxins in our homes, quietly saturating our daily lives through Wi-Fi routers, cell phones, Bluetooth wearables, cordless (DECT) phones, tablets, baby monitors, smart TVs, "smart" meters, and even nearby antennas. Unlike sunlight or X-rays, these everyday signals are *non-ionizing* radiofrequency (RF) that affect humans on a cellular level.

The International Agency for Research on Cancer (IARC) has already classified RF EMF as a Group 2B "possible carcinogen."[20] Recent research raises additional concern: One prospective study found correlations between higher household RF levels and lower scores in infant gross motor skills, fine motor skills, and problem-solving.[21] The risks rise with concentration and proximity, and common sense tells us that saturating a developing child (or a pregnant mother!) with nonstop RF signals can be detrimental.

Perhaps the clearest example of overexposure is how we carry our phones. One of the most painful trends to witness is how normalized it has become to wear or rest a phone directly on the body. Women sliding phones into bras or pregnant mothers balancing devices on their bellies like trays may not realize they are placing the most delicate and vital tissues directly in the path of concentrated emissions. Cell phone manufacturers quietly note in fine print that devices should be kept a small distance away from the body to meet federal safety standards.

Experts champion a wired-first approach at home, especially for pregnancy, infants, and children. Attorney and safe-tech advocate Odette Wilkens, Chair & General Counsel of the National Call for Safe Technology, frames it this way: *"Wired is for stationary use, and wireless is for mobility. It should not be for fixed use."* Building your home around this simple rule shrinks ambient RF without sacrificing connectivity, and it can be the single biggest step a household takes to reclaim a healthier, lower-toxin environment.[22]

Commonsense swaps:
- Hardwire computers and TVs whenever possible
- Turn Wi-Fi off at night
- Avoid wearing phones on the body
- Use speakerphone or wired air-tube headsets
- Don't sleep next to your router, smart meter, or phone
- Ditch your microwave

Even when we reduce unnecessary exposure, EMR remains an unavoidable part of modern life. One of the most powerful ways to help the body adapt is grounding, making direct contact with the earth through bare feet on grass, soil, or sand, or by using grounding mats indoors. Studies suggest grounding stabilizes the body's electrical activity, reduces inflammation, supports circadian rhythms, and may buffer the stress load created by environmental EMR. If wireless radiation is one of the invisible stressors of modern life, grounding is one of the most visible and tangible antidotes.

Your body is electrical. Treat it accordingly.

Don't Wait on the Government to Protect You

Governments are finally catching up to science: lawmakers in multiple states are now targeting PFAS and other toxic chemicals in food packaging, cookware, and storage as a public health priority. In September 2024, the federal Keep Food Containers Safe from PFAS Act (H.R. 9864) was introduced, aiming to ban intentionally added PFAS in food packaging by January 1, 2025. But in the absence of comprehensive federal action, state legislatures are leading the way: at least thirteen states, including California, Colorado, New York, and Washington, have enacted laws prohibiting intentionally added PFAS in food containers, and more than fifteen additional bills are pending. For instance, California's Safer Food Packaging Act (AB 1148) would ban bisphenols and phthalates from food packaging by 2027, while New York has extended its "forever chemical" bans beyond paper packaging to cookware and food storage, but implementation remains piecemeal, prompting environmental advocates to call this a Whac-A-Mole strategy.

This surge in regulatory attention underscores a critical message: how and where you store your food matters, not just what you put in your meals. Glass, stainless steel, and PFASfree ceramics are rapidly gaining favor, not just for their kitchen durability, but for offering real, legally backed protection against chemical leaching. As more state laws come online, these flips in policy demonstrate that consumer demand for safer food storage isn't just trendy, it's fast becoming the standard.

What We Do Next

Your ability to handle toxins depends on how well your nervous system can adapt. But when your spine is out of alignment, that adaptation breaks down. Communication between your brain and body becomes strained. Stress builds. Energy suffers.

That's where we go next. In the next chapter, you'll uncover the missing piece that keeps your nervous system stuck, and how restoring alignment can unlock the vitality that's been there all along.

CHAPTER 13

The Structural Sabotage

Look well to the spine for the cause of disease
—Hippocrates

We've started with the premise that you are designed for health, longevity, and vitality. We've established that your overall health depends on a well-functioning nervous system. We've already looked at how toxins and thoughts can create stress on that system. But there's one source of interference that's often ignored by conventional Medicine and overlooked even in natural health circles.

It's not chemical. It's not emotional. It's physical. A structural insult to the very system that keeps you alive. This form of interference doesn't come from the outside in, it comes from the inside out. And it affects how your brain communicates with your body. This kind of interference often begins subtly and often, in infancy or childhood.

Birth is one of the most powerful and miraculous human experiences. It's the moment where new life enters the world, and where a child's God-given potential hits another gear. But at the very same time, it is also one of the most physically demanding and potentially traumatic events that humans experience.

Even in a smooth, natural birth, the forces exerted on a baby's fragile spine and delicate brain stem are immense. Add to that the staggering rates of birth interventions today—C-sections, forceps, vacuum extraction, epidurals, labor induction, and more—and we see how easy it is for that miracle to be marked by trauma.

Fast-forward from birth through the years of childhood sports injuries, the thousands of hours hunched over a desk, to the "minor" car accident you walked away from without a second thought. These moments seem small, but they cause lasting changes to the spine, which is the structural and neurological foundation of your body.

When the spine shifts out of its normal alignment, even slightly, it can irritate the nervous system from within. That misalignment is called *subluxation*,[1] and it's far more than a back issue. It's a disruption in the body's communication system.

The Spine: The Lifeline Protector

Your spine isn't just a structural column keeping you upright. It is the armor protecting the most vital system in your body, the nervous system. Your brain is the command center, and your spinal cord is the information highway, carrying life-sustaining signals to every organ, tissue, and cell. If that highway is disrupted, so is communication, function, and vitality.

Think about this: If your loved one were temporarily on life support after a bad accident, and there was only one cord supplying power to keep them alive, you would expect that cord to be heavily protected. You'd expect it to be a thick, reinforced, high-durability cable because inside that cord is the power that determines the difference between life and death.

Your spine serves the same purpose. In the same way that the rubber around a power cord protects the power supply, your spine surrounds your spinal cord to protect your body's power supply. Your nervous system is the lifeline of every function in your body, and it's safeguarded by twenty-four individual, movable vertebrae that encase and protect the brain stem, spinal cord, and nerve pathways. But when these vertebrae shift out of their proper alignment, even slightly, they create interference in the nervous system. That misalignment is called subluxation.

Subluxation isn't a stiff neck or a sore back, it's a neurological disturbance that affects the way your brain and body communicate. The very word "subluxation" comes from the Latin roots: "sub" meaning "less" and "lux" meaning "light." In other words, subluxation literally means "less than light." That's exactly what it does to your nervous system. It dims the signal, reducing your body's ability to function at full capacity.

Contributor Spotlight: Dr. Tony Ebel

To deepen this chapter, we invited a voice we deeply respect in the field of neurodevelopment and pediatric chiropractic care: Dr. Tony Ebel. As the founder of the PX Docs network and a leading expert in pediatric neurology and birth trauma, Dr. Ebel brings years of clinical experience in helping children and families overcome the neurological effects of structural interference. His perspective on how early life stress and misalignment shape a child's future health adds critical weight to this chapter—and expands the vision for what's possible when we restore the spine and nervous system from the start.

Dr. Tony's Story: Oliver's Traumatic Birth and Miracle Recovery

I'm not writing this from theory. My wife and I lived it.

Our son Oliver was born about six weeks early and via a very fast, chaotic birth, he was transported from one hospital to another in ambulance. Then his condition worsened so quickly and significantly, he was life-flighted in a helicopter to yet another hospital. Eventually he would require a heart-lung bypass procedure called ECMO to help his tiny little heart and lungs heal, and multiple other surgeries as well over the course of a six-week NICU stay.

Oliver is a medical miracle, as we were blessed to see the best of the modern medical machine. In crisis, emergency, urgent care Medicine is truly life-saving and incredible. However, once they "put the fire out" and we knew Oliver was going to live, the prognosis was as grave and dim as it gets.

The Harvard trained neurologist informed us that if he lived past the age of one, he had a "99 percent chance" of struggling with severe cerebral palsy, epilepsy, and autism due to his significant hypoxic brain injury at birth. The news they delivered made sense because his EEG and MRI findings were awful.

However, we knew from the start that Oliver would be different. We knew that God designed us all to heal, especially children. And we knew that He put that healing power within the nervous system, and gave us chiropractic care to adjust subluxations, clear interference, and activate the healing process from the inside out like no drug, surgery, or other intervention can.

I adjusted Oliver two to three times per day, every single day for those six weeks. Each time, we'd work to calm his overactive sympathetic nervous system and stimulate his suppressed vagus nerve and parasympathetic system—the healing, repair, and regulation side of life.

While I did so, we'd watch on the monitors as his blood pressure would come down, breathing rate normalize, and pulse ox numbers go up—which were beyond essential for him since his primary condition was persistent pulmonary hypertension (PPHN) and the resultant hypoxic brain injury.

What looked like structural care on the outside, was really life-changing nervous system–focused care on the inside!

Oliver would end up leaving the hospital at the end of that six weeks with his miracle already revealed! His seizures gone, respiratory struggles gone, nervous system distress gone, digestion improved, respiratory rate normalized, and so much more. He was off all medications and not only that, his EEG and MRI were fully clear, giving us direct evidence of his brain and nervous system healing.

Oliver's recovery was a mystery to the medical team. They termed it "spontaneous recovery" and just moved on to the next case. That's okay, one day they'll understand that God put the true potential of healing within our nervous system, and those of us doctors who can access it and support it with hands alone instead of drugs will be the ones positioned firmly where we need to be in all of pediatric and family healthcare—as the foundation.

To this day, Oliver's story is the most powerful testimony I could ever give about the devastating effects of subluxation—and the miraculous potential for healing when it is corrected and adjusted!

Every parent deserves to know that birth trauma is real, that subluxation is common, and that there is a safe, effective way to help their child heal and thrive. Every child deserves to start life not with structural sabotage, but with nervous system regulation and optimization!

Our family lived through the dark side of birth trauma, but we also got to experience the miraculous side of neurological healing! Oliver's story proves that when we remove interference and restore connection, miracles happen!

Birth Trauma: The First Misalignment

Oliver's story is not unique. Research and clinical experience both show that nearly all infants experience some degree of birth trauma to the spine and nervous system. In a study of 1,250 infants evaluated within the first five days of life, it was found that 90 percent had suffered birth trauma and strain in the neck and cranial areas, with 10 percent suffering severe trauma.[2] Another study examining 1,000 infants in their first month of life found that 80 percent had vertebral misalignment in the upper neck.[3] Modern research shows that even births without obvious complications can damage the cervical spine, and spinal cord injury contributes to roughly 10 percent of neonatal deaths.[4]

The studies done in the mid- to late twentieth century are informative but conservative. Over the past decades, there's been a dramatic shift in delivery methods: vacuum-assisted births now account for 10–15 percent of vaginal deliveries, and C-sections have surged from under 7 percent in the 1970s to over 30 percent in recent years.[5] These assisted deliveries—while lifesaving—apply significant mechanical forces across a newborn's spine and neck. Many studies report 80–90 percent showing misalignment or biomechanical stress in the upper spine within days of delivery.[6]

Nearly every newborn enters life with some degree of spinal strain. And yet, unless their parents have a relationship with a neurospinal and pediatric-trained chiropractor, these misalignments go unchecked. Left uncorrected, these early subluxations can alter nervous system function, affect digestion, sleep, and immune resilience, and set the stage for chronic issues later in life. Birth trauma isn't just a possibility, it's become the norm. And it's one of the most overlooked factors in early childhood health.

Pain Is a Poor Indicator of Health

Here's what most people don't realize: Subluxation doesn't always cause pain. In fact, it usually doesn't. Only a small portion of the nervous system is dedicated to pain perception, while the majority of the nervous system is responsible for essential functions, like organ regulation, sensory processing and motor control. This is why you can have significant spinal misalignment and neurological interference without ever experiencing pain.

Think about it, does high blood pressure hurt? Does diabetes in its early stages cause pain? No. But by the time symptoms show up, the body has already been compensating for dysfunction for years. Waiting for pain to tell you something is wrong is like waiting for your car engine to seize up before checking the oil. When your spine is misaligned, it doesn't always create discomfort, but it always creates dysfunction. And dysfunction is the first step toward disease.

Why This Matters More than You Think

Let's just address it now. I'm a chiropractor telling you about the importance of addressing spinal misalignments. You might expect me to say that. But this isn't about chiropractic care. This is about understanding the undeniable reality that your nervous system controls every function in your body and the importance of spinal alignment.

You can eat all the right foods, exercise daily, and take every supplement on the shelf, but if your nervous system is stuck in stress mode, none of that will make the impact you're looking for. From over a decade of firsthand experience, the game change is when we shift how your brain and body communicate. That's when metabolism resets, inflammation drops, and your body finally starts to heal the way it was designed to.

The encouraging part about taking care of your spine and nervous system is that it increases your ability to adapt to all of the unavoidable stressors on our brains and bodies. Anxieties, migraines, behavioral issues, mental health issues, cancers, and even fertility issues are all examples of the body's inability to adapt and heal in its environment. Yes, it is always a good idea to clean up known offenders in your environment by removing known toxins, etc., but it is even more important to be able to adapt to modern life, from demands at work, parenting, and being in relationship to the invisible toxins like cell phone radiation. When we support our bodies' innate ability to heal and remove subluxations, we can restore confidence that we are capable of adapting.

Map of the Spine

It might surprise you to hear about the spine's connection with the nervous system, as Oliver's story illustrates. But at every level of your spine, nerves exit and travel to specific organs and systems. You've probably seen those posters in medical offices, the ones that show how each spinal level is linked to a specific organ.

The nerves that exit the spine communicate with various systems. The upper neck can influence the eyes, ears, and thyroid. The mid-back connects with the lungs, heart, and stomach. The lower back impacts the bladder, bowels, and reproductive organs.

But here's where we go deeper. Subluxation doesn't just affect a single nerve going to a single part of the body. That view is too mechanical and too limited. When your spine shifts out of alignment, it changes the tone of the entire nervous system. It sends danger signals to the brain, activates stress pathways, and flips your body into a fight-or-flight state, even when there is no real threat.

That means digestion slows down. Hormones become imbalanced. Immune function weakens. And energy is rerouted away from healing and toward survival. Subluxation does not just interfere with nerve flow. It alters the brain's perception of safety. And that changes everything.

The Brain Effects of Subluxation

Research by Dr. Heidi Haavik has shown that spinal misalignment changes the way the brain processes sensory information. When subluxation is present, it disrupts proprioception (your body's ability to sense and control movement), leading to dysfunctional movement patterns, postural instability, and an overactive stress response.[7]

Even more significant is how subluxation affects the prefrontal cortex, the part of your brain responsible for decision-making, emotional regulation, autonomic function, and coordination. When the spine is out of alignment, it alters neural input to this region, keeping the body locked in a state of stress and dysfunction.[8]

This is why subluxation isn't just about pain. It's about neurological interference that keeps your body from healing properly. Left uncorrected, it can contribute to chronic stress, metabolic dysfunction, pain sensitivity, and poor immune regulation.

Research has demonstrated that subluxation leads to measurable physiological consequences:

- **Negative neuroplastic and autonomic changes**—Subluxation alters neural pathways, reinforcing chronic stress and disrupting autonomic balance.[9]
- **Decreased brain stem and/or brain blood flow**—Misalignment, particularly in the upper cervical spine, has been linked to reduced cerebral perfusion, impacting cognitive function and nervous system regulation.[10]
- **Increased inflammation**—Chronic spinal dysfunction contributes to systemic inflammation, which is linked to pain, metabolic disorders, and even neurodegenerative diseases.[11]
- **Cerebrospinal fluid alterations**—Structural issues in the spine can impair the natural flow of cerebrospinal fluid, increasing intracranial pressure and leading to neurological symptoms.[12]
- **Mechanical spinal cord tension**—Misalignment creates unnecessary tension on the spinal cord, affecting nerve transmission and overall function.[13]

Jay's Story

Jay came to our office exhausted and skeptical. He had tried everything, anti-inflammatories, digestive aids, antipsychotics but nothing touched the fatigue, brain fog, and migraines that were wrecking his daily life. What changed his trajectory wasn't another pill, it was identifying and correcting subluxation. We found a major misalignment in his upper cervical spine, one that had likely been there since childhood. After a few months of specific neurospinal correction and restoring proper alignment, Jay's sleep returned, energy restored, and the fog lifted. He got his life back, not because we treated his migraines or chased his symptoms, but because we restored the communication between his brain and body.

Subluxation creates an environment where your body is constantly fighting against itself, stuck in a loop of stress, tension, and dysfunction.

And unless it's corrected, no amount of exercise, nutrition, or supplements will fully restore your vitality.

A Line in the Sand: Recognizing the Need for a Structural Shift

Before we move into the real solutions in part 3, you need to ask yourself a crucial question: Who is protecting your nervous system? If you don't have a neurospinal corrective chiropractor in your corner, you're leaving the most vital system in your body unprotected. Given what we now know about the nervous system, this isn't optional. If your spine is compromised, your health is compromised. Period.

In the next section, we will dive into the strategies to rebuild and restore the gut. But before you can truly move forward, you have to acknowledge that the modern world has set a trap, and most people are walking right into it. Your family's spine and nervous system have taken a hit. The question is, will you let the abuse continue?

CHAPTER 14

Gut Health and the Microbiome Connection

Twenty-four hours a day, seven days a week, our GI tract, enteric nervous system, and brain are in constant communication.
—Emeran Mayer, *The Mind-Gut Connection*

Your gut isn't just breaking down food, it's calling the shots for your entire body. It controls immune defense, brain function, metabolism, and inflammation. When your gut is thriving, so are you. But when it's off balance, the effects ripple through every system, setting the stage for dysfunction and disease.

This isn't just about bloating or acid reflux. A dysfunctional gut is the silent driver behind autoimmune disorders, hormonal imbalances, and chronic inflammation.[1] It dictates whether your brain is sharp or foggy, whether your metabolism hums or stalls, and whether your immune system is resilient or overwhelmed. Your gut health determines whether you're building vitality or breaking down.

If you're struggling with fatigue, brain fog, or chronic health issues, your gut is likely sending you a message. The problem is, most people don't recognize the signs until they're deep in dysfunction. The good news? You can turn it around. The gut is incredibly adaptive, and when you remove the insults and give it what it needs, it rebuilds, rebalances, and restores vitality from the inside out.

I've lived this firsthand. Let me take you back to the beginning of my own gut healing journey. I shared this briefly in the introduction but there's an additional layer that is appropriate here.

Nick's Story: From Peak Fitness to Falling Apart

I wasn't your typical "gut patient." At eighteen, I looked like I had it all dialed in: clear skin, lean muscle, 6 percent body fat. I lived in the gym. I ate clean, or at least what I thought was clean. From the outside, I looked like the picture of health. But inside, I was spiraling.

At first it was just a little bloating. Then urgency. Then I was sprinting to the bathroom five to ten times a day. Blood in the toilet became normal. Doctors ran some tests, shrugged, and labeled it: *Inflammatory Bowel Disease*. They handed me prescriptions and moved on.

I wasn't okay with that. By the world's standards, I was "doing everything right." But I wasn't healing. It wasn't until I was introduced to a doctor who practiced true natural health that things finally changed.

I stopped treating symptoms and started rebuilding my body. I changed my inputs. I cleaned up my food, cleared out toxins, started regular chiropractic care, and used targeted supplements to support my gut lining and microbiome. That year, my symptoms not only improved but more importantly, I learned a deeper truth: healing is a state of being, not a finish line. And the gut isn't optional, it's foundational.

Your gut isn't just about digestion, it's the domino piece that tips everything else in motion. If mine could break down despite everything I thought I was doing "right," it's worth asking: *what else have we misunderstood about gut health?*

The Gut and Microbiome: The Heart of Healing

If you want to reclaim your vitality, your gut has to be part of the plan. Inside you is an entire ecosystem, a living network of trillions of bacteria, fungi, and other microbes, each with a job to do.[2] Some help break down food, extracting the nutrients that fuel your cells. Others regulate your immune system, acting as the frontline defense against invaders. Some even manufacture neurotransmitters, shaping your mood, memory, and mental resilience.

The balance of your microbiome isn't just important, it's essential to adapting to external stressors and supporting daily healing. When it's thriving, your body absorbs nutrients efficiently, your immune system reacts appropriately, and your brain operates at full capacity. But when it's out of balance? The effects ripple through every system. Nutrient deficiencies creep in. Inflammation spikes. The immune system becomes confused, overreacting to harmless substances and triggering autoimmune conditions. Brain fog, anxiety, and fatigue take hold. These are all signals and reg flags that your microbiome is damaged, disrupted and asking for help to restore the symbiosis among your microbiota. Below we explore the most common causes of a disrupted microbiome and inflamed gut.

Antibiotics: The Double-Edged Sword

It's hard to discuss the gut without first addressing one of the biggest culprits that has caused such widespread gut and immune system challenges: antibiotics. Antibiotics don't just kill harmful bacteria, they carpet-bomb your microbiome, wiping out the beneficial bacteria your gut needs to function and destroying the symbiosis your body is designed to maintain. Gut bacteria should exist in harmony with the vast and diverse microbiota, but when the balance is thrown off, health problems explode. This is called dysbiosis and can be confirmed with specialty microbiome testing. And the consequences of dysbiosis are seen in the modern-day explosion of diagnoses of infertility, mental health issues, cancer, brain disease, and diabetes.[3]

Research from *Science Daily* found that those who took antibiotics for over six months had a 17 percent greater risk of developing cancer in the ascending colon compared to those who didn't.[4] The damage to the intestinal lining was still visible five to ten years later, and even a single round of antibiotics leaves a mark.[5] But the real takeaway? The balance of life is delicate, intricate, brilliant, and cannot be artificially manipulated without costly disruption. Antibiotics begin the process of disruption, fueling the path for inflammation and leakiness of the gut. Be encouraged that there is nearly always an alternative to antibiotic use. But take caution that not all alternatives are equal.

The Fire of Gut Inflammation: What's Fueling the Blaze?

Inflammation has long been demonized. So it is important to understand and respect that inflammation is the body's natural defense mechanism. When you get a cut, your immune system kicks in, sending in white blood cells to fight infection and heal the wound. That's normal, that's necessary. But when inflammation becomes chronic, when the body never stops fighting, damage spreads like wildfire. And nowhere is this more destructive than in the gut.

Most people think gut inflammation is something you can "cool down" with a turmeric capsule and call it a day. That's not how this works. You can't put out a fire while you're still stoking the coals. If you don't stop the underlying assault that causes the body to intelligently inflame, no amount of anti-inflammatories (even natural ones) will resolve your issues. The real question is: what's fueling the fire in the first place? The approach to healing is not to "control" inflammation, but instead to listen to the body, identify the fuel source, and *make changes* so that you can watch the inflammation reduce signaling resolve. How else would you watch for resolution and have assurance that the body has returned to a state of repair?

The Root Causes of Gut Inflammation

Inflammation doesn't happen in a vacuum. It's a direct reaction to constant irritation, an immune system on high alert because something is repeatedly attacking it. The good news is that there are six common culprits that we can expose and eliminating those culprits creates a big shift in healing and an accelerated understanding going forward.

- **Processed Foods and Refined Sugars**—These aren't food; they're food-like substances, chemical weapons against your gut. They feed harmful bacteria, trigger insulin resistance, and keep your immune system in a constant state of stress.[6] All of these effects are detrimental to your primary functions as a human. This is not about being a "health nut." It's about awareness and knowledge of what should go into your body. Added sugars and artificial sugars saturate these products. Preservatives and stabilizers are unavoidable for shelf stability. And the industry standards are no assurance of "safe" consumption because their reference point is so far off. Make no mistake: there are things on the shelves that are destructive to your body. A constant drip of unnatural, chemical substances is devastating to your system.

- **Bad Fats (a.k.a. Processed Seed Oils)**—*Canola, soybean, corn, cottonseed, vegetable, sunflower and safflower* oils are everywhere, hidden in restaurant meals, packaged foods, and even so-called "health foods." They oxidize easily, create free radicals (think cancer-causing), and fuel inflammation like dry wood to a flame. Fat got a bad rap for cholesterol and heart issues. But not all fats are equal. Bad fats are responsible for more than heart disease. They are a main driver of overall inflammation in your body. And good fats are not the enemy, they are absolutely necessary for brain health and cellular function.[7] Therefore it is critical that you distinguish between bad fats and good fats.

- **Gluten and Denatured Dairy**—If your gut is compromised, these proteins act like tiny knives, stabbing at and permeating the intestinal lining. The more damage, the more inflammation, and the cycle continues. If you have been vaccinated, taken antibiotics, or eaten conventional produce or grains, then your gut is likely compromised to some extent. So sadly, this applies to most people. Gluten is a complex topic but is undoubtedly a primary culprit behind gut inflammation.

- **Toxins, Pesticides, and Heavy Metals**—Every day, you're exposed to environmental toxins that disrupt gut bacteria and trigger immune responses through public water, air, food, and even personal care products. Yes, all of those things affect the gut. Glyphosate (a widely used herbicide found in conventional grains, legumes, and even some organic ones) is particularly dangerous, wiping out beneficial bacteria and making the gut more permeable.[8] Glyphosate carpet-bombs beneficial microbes that are essential for digestion, immune regulation, and the production of vital nutrients provoking chronic inflammation and autoimmunity.[9] Heavy metals like mercury, lead, and arsenic further damage the gut lining and disrupt the microbial balance,[10] while pesticide residues interfere with enzyme function and hormone signaling.[11] Over time, the toxic load overwhelms the body's detoxification pathways, leaving the gut inflamed.

- **Medications (Especially Antibiotics and NSAIDs)**— Medications are one of the most overlooked contributors to gut dysfunction, especially antibiotics and NSAIDs. Antibiotics are designed to kill bacteria, but they do so indiscriminately, wiping out not only the overgrowth of certain microbes but also the diverse population of good microbes that form the foundation of a healthy gut ecosystem.[12] This microbial wipeout leaves the gut vulnerable to opportunistic infections like *C. difficile*, reduces microbial diversity, and, without intentional healing, takes years to recover. Nonsteroidal anti-inflammatory drugs (NSAIDs), such as ibuprofen pose a different but equally damaging threat. They compromise the integrity of the gut lining by inhibiting protective prostaglandins, leading to increased intestinal permeability and microscopic damage that results in chronic inflammation.[13]

- **Chronic Stress and Poor Sleep**—You could eat the cleanest diet in the world, but if your stress is through the roof and you're sleeping five hours or less a night, your gut will still suffer. Stress weakens the gut barrier, disrupts digestion, and makes inflammation worse.[14] Sleep is a gift from God that is meant to put your body into a state of peace and calm and accelerated healing at the end of each day. It is the time that we let go of control, stop solving problems, and watching the wall for dangers. Without this gift of peace and healing each night, all of our physical disrepair is perpetually exacerbated instead of divinely resolved. Peace and sleep are nonnegotiables. If these are problem spots, don't give up on getting to the bottom of it.

The Consequences of an Inflamed Gut

This isn't just about bloating or bellyaches. An inflamed gut can quietly wreak havoc across your entire body. When inflammation damages the intestinal lining, it creates tiny openings that allow undigested food particles, toxins, and microbes to enter the bloodstream. This breach, often called "leaky gut," triggers an immune system on high alert, launching widespread inflammation that disrupts everything from mood and mental clarity to hormones, energy levels, and even fertility.[15] And here's the catch: the fallout doesn't always show up as digestive symptoms. Instead, it often surfaces where your body is most vulnerable, such as autoimmune disease, brain fog, chronic fatigue, mood disorders, or metabolic issues.[16] The longer the gut remains compromised, the more entrenched these systemic problems become, often going unrecognized until they manifest as full-blown illness.

Leaky Gut Syndrome: A Breach in the Body's Defense System?

Your gut isn't just a digestive organ, it's the front line of your immune system. It decides what gets in and what stays out, filtering nutrients while keeping pathogens and toxins at bay. But when chronic inflammation weakens the intestinal lining, this barrier breaks down. Toxins, undigested food particles, and harmful bacteria start leaking into the bloodstream, triggering an immune response that never turns off. This is leaky gut syndrome, and it's not just a digestive issue, it's a system-wide alarm bell.

But here's the key distinction: the immune system isn't attacking the body. It's responding to a crisis. The conventional model frames autoimmunity as a tragic case of "mistaken identity" of let's say a peanut, where the body turns against itself. That's a fundamental misunderstanding. Your immune system doesn't randomly go rogue. It's an intelligent, adaptive system, responding to what it perceives as a threat. If your gut is constantly leaking inflammatory particles into circulation, your immune system will respond accordingly, with chronic inflammation, tissue repair, and immune activation that can appear destructive.

Once the gut barrier is compromised, the immune system shifts into constant battle mode. It detects foreign invaders (food proteins, bacteria, toxins) and mobilizes an inflammatory response to contain the damage. But when these triggers don't stop and you keep introducing new offenders, neither does the immune response.

This isn't just about bloating or IBS. Leaky gut is a foundational driver of autoimmune conditions, neurological dysfunction, and metabolic breakdown.[17] Where the damage shows up depends on the individual, but the pattern is the same:

- If the immune system is dealing with viral reactivations or toxins stored in the joints, it presents as **rheumatoid arthritis** or **joint pain**.
- If it's constantly clearing out inflammatory food particles that mimic thyroid proteins, it shows up as **Hashimoto's thyroiditis**.
- If it's struggling with chronic gut infections and bacterial overgrowth, it manifests as **Crohn's** or **ulcerative colitis**.
- If gut-derived inflammation reaches the brain, it contributes to brain fog, anxiety, depression, and even neurodegenerative conditions like **Alzheimer's**.

This isn't the immune system attacking for no reason. It's a response to an unresolved threat, a continuous assault coming from inside the gut.

Leaky Gut: A Gateway to Autoimmune Dysfunction

Most people don't connect their joint pain, fatigue, or brain fog to gut health because the symptoms appear outside the digestive system. But this is exactly how chronic disease begins. The gut leaks inflammatory triggers into the bloodstream, and the immune system fights back wherever it sees the most damage.

The more chronic the assault, the more widespread the damage becomes. And if the root cause isn't removed, the immune system stays locked in defense mode. This is why conventional treatments that simply suppress the immune system with steroids or immunosuppressants fail, they're not addressing the fire, just silencing the alarm.

The only way forward? Seal the gut, remove the triggers, and allow the immune system to recalibrate. The body isn't broken, it's doing exactly what it was designed to do. The real question is: Are you fueling the fire, or are you putting it out? Now, let's talk about exactly how to repair a leaky gut.

The Three Steps to Healing Leaky Gut

Healing the gut isn't complicated, but it does require a strategic approach. It is imperative to stop the assault and then rebuild. The gut doesn't just heal because you take supplements. It heals when you remove the cause of damage. You can flood your system with probiotics, glutamine, and turmeric, but if you're still eating inflammatory foods, popping ibuprofen like candy, and sleeping five hours a night, you're going nowhere. There are three essential steps: Remove, Rebuild, and Replenish: a systematic way to repair the gut lining, restore microbial balance, and bring the body back to health.

Step 1: Eliminate—Remove the Offenders

The first step isn't to "add more." The first step is clearing out what's hurting you in the first place. Stop the daily assault by removing the inflammatory triggers most often found in the six common culprits at the beginning of this chapter. Identify your culprits and give your gut *the break* it needs to regenerate. Only then can you start the process of rebuilding. Be aware of the myth of "everything in moderation," because when your gut lining is damaged, even a speck of the offender keeps you stuck.

And when you do? Everything changes. Inflammation drops. Brain function sharpens. Energy skyrockets. Pain fades. It doesn't take long at all to notice the change. The gut is at the center of it all, and once you heal it, you unlock the health you were meant to have.

For many, the biggest culprits are hidden food sensitivities, with gluten and glyphosate-laden grains being some of the worst offenders. These trigger an immune response that keeps the gut in a constant state of attack. Removing inflammatory foods allows the gut lining to stop reacting and begin the repair process. During this phase, antimicrobial herbs, fasting, and detox support can help eliminate harmful bacteria, yeast overgrowth, and gut pathogens that have taken over. It's also advised to incorporate a full spectrum of digestive enzymes as a support during all three phases of gut healing.

Step 2: Repair—Rebuild the Gut Lining

Once the gut is no longer under constant assault, it's time to rebuild. The gut lining regenerates quickly when given the right tools, nutrients that restore the integrity of the intestinal barrier.

L-glutamine, collagen, and immunoglobulins are key players here. These compounds act like bricks and mortar, sealing up the gaps in the gut lining and strengthening its defenses.[18] Bone broth, rich in amino acids and gelatin, helps restore elasticity and resilience.[19] Meanwhile, anti-inflammatory compounds like curcumin, aloe vera, and omega-3s calm the fire that has been burning for too long.[20]

Rebuilding the gut also means supporting digestion. If stomach acid is too low, food won't break down properly, leading to bloating, nutrient malabsorption, and bacterial overgrowth.[21] I recommend adding organic apple cider vinegar (ACV) with the digestive enzymes to help restore proper breakdown and absorption of food.

Like with anything, the components you employ to rebuild matter. Make sure you are using quality sources without additives or artificial ingredients.

Step 3: Replenish—Reinoculate the Microbiome

With the gut lining restored, the final step is replenishing the microbiome. This means reintroducing the beneficial bacteria that keep digestion, immunity, and metabolism in check. A healthy microbiome is like a thriving forest, lush, diverse, and teeming with synergistic life. It's home to trillions of bacteria, fungi, and other microorganisms, *each* playing a unique role in maintaining balance, harmony, and resilience within your body. In this vibrant inner ecosystem, every microbe plays a role. Some break down food, some extract nutrients, some produce essential vitamins like B_{12} and K_2, and some even generate neurotransmitters like serotonin and dopamine that influence your mood.[22]

When your microbiome is in balance, digestion feels smooth and effortless, energy flows steadily, the mind is clear, and inflammation is a tool used to resolve acute situations. Healing the gut isn't just about manipulating "good" and "bad," it is about nurturing the complex and innately brilliant internal ecosystem that self-governs and self-heals.

A diverse, fiber-rich diet filled with prebiotics and probiotics, such as lacto-fermented foods like sauerkraut, kimchi, kefir, and bitter yogurt (no sugar or sugar substitutes), feeds the beneficial microbes that keep the gut balanced.[23] Probiotics from quality supplements can assist in repopulating the gut with healthy strains. Spore-based probiotics, which survive stomach acid and thrive in the intestines, are particularly powerful in gut restoration.

Replenishing doesn't stop with probiotics. A healthy gut thrives on diversity, with exposure to different types of bacteria from regenerative-organic soil and fermented foods. The goal isn't just to add good bacteria but to create an environment where they can thrive long-term.

Leaky Brain

Your gut and brain are constantly in conversation, linked by the vagus nerve and chemical messengers that shape everything from mood to memory.[24] The vagus nerve is the body's communication superhighway, carrying messages between the brain and gut in both directions. It helps regulate digestion, inflammation, mood, and even heart rate.

When gut bacteria are thriving, neurotransmitters like serotonin and dopamine fire on all cylinders, keeping your mind sharp and your emotions stable. But when dysbiosis sets in? Anxiety, depression, brain fog, and even neurodegenerative diseases can take root.[25]

Just as your gut has a protective lining that keeps harmful substances out of the bloodstream, your brain is shielded by what's called the blood-brain barrier, a specialized wall of tightly packed cells designed to prevent toxins, pathogens, and inflammatory compounds from entering delicate brain tissue. But this barrier, like the gut lining, can become compromised. When it does, it allows substances that don't belong, such as inflammatory cytokines, environmental toxins, and even bacterial fragments, to seep into the brain. This is what researchers are now calling *leaky brain*, a condition linked to cognitive decline, anxiety, depression, brain fog, and even neurodegenerative diseases like Alzheimer's.[26]

From a vitalistic perspective, the body is an interconnected, intelligent system designed to heal and maintain balance. When inflammation takes root in the gut and the microbiome is disrupted, the ripple effect reaches far beyond digestion. In fact, the gut and the brain are in constant communication through the vagus nerve, the immune system, and chemical messengers like neurotransmitters. This relationship is so powerful that the gut is often called the "second brain." So when the gut becomes inflamed or leaky, the blood-brain barrier often follows suit, breaking down under the same systemic inflammatory load and allowing damaging substances to cross into the brain's protected space.

The signs of a leaky brain can be subtle at first, such as difficulty concentrating, forgetfulness, mental fatigue, and irritability, but over time they can evolve into serious neurological and psychiatric conditions that cannot be healed by assigning it a label and taking a psychiatric drug. Yet instead of recognizing this as a call to restore internal harmony, conventional Medicine often rushes to silence symptoms with more medications, which may further disrupt the gut-brain axis.[27] A vitalistic approach sees these signs not as isolated problems, but as signals, intelligent alerts from the body that something deeper needs attention. Healing begins not with suppression, but with restoration: rebuilding the gut lining, supporting detoxification, calming the nervous system, and nurturing the microbiome.

True brain health cannot be separated from gut health. By reducing

---

The Power of Microbiome Testing

The gut doesn't lie. A stool test is more than just a snapshot of bacteria, it can be an inside look at how well your gut is handling digestion, immunity, and inflammation. These tests can reveal bacterial imbalances, hidden infections, and inflammatory markers that tell the real story of your health. Understanding your microbiome means you can take precise action, fixing what's broken and restoring what's missing. If you're serious about gut health, it starts with knowing exactly what's happening inside. The microbiome is the gatekeeper of many systems, and when it's in balance, the body thrives. But when it's neglected, disease takes hold. The good news? You have the power to change it. Every bite, every habit, every choice either fuels dysfunction or fosters resilience.

If you're ready to take the first step, we recommend advanced microbiome tests for our patients. You can learn more and order it directly by visiting Dr-Wilson.com/Tests.

toxic burden, nourishing beneficial microbes, and rebuilding the intestinal lining, we also begin to reseal the brain's protective barrier. In this way, healing becomes holistic. It's not just about preventing disease; it's about creating an internal environment where clarity, focus, and emotional resilience can thrive. The body, when supported, always moves toward wholeness. The gut drives the brain. Get this system right, and many other dominoes fall correctly.

Hopefully by now you can visualize the possibility of continual healing and adaptation. The paradigm shift from being at the mercy of Medicine to vitality, happens through knowledge and through action. Parts 1 and 2 were all about acquiring knowledge to exit Medicine and live naturally. In part 3, we'll move from theory to practice, laying out a clear road map to build vitality, from the ground up. This is where vitality stops being an idea and health freedom takes root.

PART III

Experience Health Freedom

Principle 1: Your body was designed to heal.
Principle 2: The Body Can Become Devitalized.
Principle 3: **Every Solution Must Align with Revitalization.**

Principle 3 isn't just an idea, it's the guiding principle you use to measure every health decision you make. If a solution doesn't restore vitality, it isn't solving the problem. It's masking it. And every time you suppress a symptom instead of addressing its root cause, you take a step further from true health rather than toward it, which prolongs the healing journey, can create unnecessary suffering, and often has a cascade effect that leads to more and more intervention. You can see the cycle.

This part of the book is about reclaiming your birthright: health freedom. Not just the freedom to make choices about your health, but the freedom to build health, true, thriving, unapologetic vitality. One of the biggest differences between this approach and Medicine is the belief that you *can* heal and that you *do* have options.

Health freedom begins with a nervous system that's fully alive.

Sadly, most people are stuck in survival mode, chronically inflamed, overcommitted, under-recovered, mentally strung out, and chasing the next protocol. They've tried diets, workouts, biohacks, and supplements, but they're still exhausted. That's not a discipline problem. It's a nervous system regulation problem.

This is your new road map. The chapters ahead will walk you through the "how to's" to reclaim vitality. This layered strategy is designed to retrain your nervous system, restore function, and rebuild resilience. The chapters

179

ahead will take you beyond theory and into action. This is how we reclaim health as individuals and together as a community, not by managing or fighting decline, but by rewiring the body to heal. The cultural shift that awaits is revolutionary.

CHAPTER 15

The Seven Virtues of a Vitalist: The Pursuit of Mastery

It is easier to prevent bad habits than to break them.

—Benjamin Franklin

Leah and I were standing in line at the coffee shop when a young man in front of me grabbed two cans of Pepsi, turned around and recognizing me, he said, "This probably isn't healthy, is it?"

I smiled. I have had this same exchange more times than I can count. Several years ago, I walked up to the checkout at the grocery store to find a patient unloading Pop-Tarts and orange-colored soda onto the conveyor belt. She laughed and said, "We don't normally eat like this." Other times, I'd be at lunch with someone who "accidentally" ordered the unhealthy item and "begrudgingly" ate it anyway.

Leah gets a kick out of these moments. When we were first married, her grandfather gave me a simple rule: we do not discuss nutrition at the dinner table. I learned that lesson the hard way after giving a mini health lecture over Sunday lunch. He smiled and gently said, "Nick, we don't discuss nutrition at the dinner table."

So I don't bring up nutrition at mealtime anymore. But inevitably, it finds its way into these moments, exemplified by the young man asking, "This probably isn't healthy, is it?

Here is the truth: people do not change because they know something.

They change because they believe something. Information does not transform lives. Conviction does.

The Loma Linda Example

Until information is connected to a deep and compelling philosophy or virtue, it rarely produces change. Consider the Blue Zones, the regions studied by Dan Buettner where people live the longest, healthiest lives on earth. The only Blue Zone in the United States, Loma Linda, is home to a large population of Seventh-day Adventists in Southern California.

They live longer not because they discovered a new supplement or a trending diet, but because their belief system reinforces their behavior. They eat clean, rest habitually, spend time in community, and honor God through their stewardship of the body. Their health is not accidental. It is the by-product of living with conviction.

That brings us to an important principle. Most people believe that once they *have* health, they will finally be able to *do* the things healthy people do and eventually *become* healthy. They wait for results to change identity.

But life does not work that way. You must first *be* the kind of person who values health as a virtue. Then you will naturally *do* what a healthy person does. Only then will you *have* the fruit of vitality.

The order matters. Identity precedes action, and action produces results. The mistake most people make is trying to reverse that order, thinking discipline or motivation will carry them. But without virtue, without becoming, their doing fades and their having never lasts.

Vitality begins with *being*. Be a Vitalist first. No matter what doctors have told you about your genetics, family history, and what diagnosis you've received, you can be a Vitalist. If there's life in your bones, you too can be a Vitalist.

What It Means to Be a Vitalist

A Vitalist is someone who believes that life is not random or mechanical, but divinely designed and intelligently ordered. A Vitalist sees the body not as a machine to be managed, but as a living system capable of self-healing, adaptation, and renewal.

To be a Vitalist is to reject the idea that health is the absence of disease or the product of modern medicine. It is to recognize that health is the natural state of a body that is aligned with truth.

A Vitalist honors the laws of life, the same natural and moral laws that govern the mind, body, and spirit. A Vitalist takes responsibility for cultivating those conditions, not through fear or control, but through stewardship and virtue.

Being a Vitalist is not about perfection. It is the daily pursuit of order in the midst of chaos, peace in the presence of stress, and conviction in the face of convenience.

So before you *do* the work of health, you must decide who you will *be*. Be a person who lives from virtue, acts from conviction, and you will have the life your design intended. You'll *be* a Vitalist.

So what separates those who simply believe in vitality from those who truly live it? The answer is virtue. Belief without practice creates a divided life, one where your mind knows the truth, but your habits tell a different story.

The Vitalist's task is to close that gap. To bring the body, the mind, and the spirit into alignment so that conviction becomes action and truth becomes behavior. That is where virtue enters the picture. Virtue is the bridge between what you know and what you live.

The Case for Virtue

When someone says, "I know this isn't good for me, but I'm going to do it anyway," that is not a lack of information. They already know the apple is better than the donut. The problem is not ignorance; it is incongruence. The gap between knowing and doing is enormous, and most people fall into it daily.

That gap is what this chapter is about: the space between information and transformation.

You have spent the first part of this book learning how the body heals and the systems that support vitality. But to sustain it, you need more than knowledge. You need conviction. You need virtue.

Benjamin Franklin understood this. At age twenty, he began a personal experiment to master himself. He created a list of thirteen virtues such as temperance, order, resolution, and humility, and tracked his progress daily. He was not obsessed with perfection. He was devoted to practice. He knew that the good life was not achieved by chance but through disciplined pursuit. This is a mind-blowing recognition to most people when it comes to their health. Medicine has convinced everyone that health is random chance and bad luck. That simply isn't true.

The heart of the Vitalist journey is to live by principle, to master the body by mastering the self, and to align your health with your values and your values with virtue.

The Seven Virtues of a Vitalist are not habits to check off a list. They are standards to aspire to. Each one builds foundational strength and when applied, physiological resilience. Together, they form the backbone of a life of vitality. I can promise you that the results from adopting these standards are not a distant thought in the future. You will be amazed at how quickly you notice changes, and sometimes big changes, fast.

The Seven Virtues of a Vitalist

1. **Mental fortitude**—Guard your thoughts and renew your mind continually.
2. **Clean living**—Refuse what is toxic and choose what gives life.
3. **Food temperance**—Fast regularly and live free.
4. **Movement**—Stay in motion; life flows through action.
5. **Alignment**—Strengthen your structure and live aligned with purpose.
6. **Nonintervention**—Limit outside-in treatments; allow healing from within.
7. **Rest**—Protect and honor deep sleep and restorative rhythms.

Each virtue represents a pillar of vitality. You already know how the body restores and heals. You have seen how the nervous system controls and coordinates every function. Now it is time to live those truths out.

A brain that holds knowledge while a body acts in contradiction will always produce frustration. The goal is not perfection but pursuit.

Defined virtues bring coherence to every dimension of your health–mind, body and spirit.

The Vitality Balance Sheet

That brings us to the practical side of this pursuit: knowing where you stand today. Franklin kept his ledger of virtues to track his progress. You will do something similar. But instead of tracking pride and humility, you will track markers of vitality and depletion. This exercise will help you see reality clearly, without judgment or shame, and it will reveal where your energy, time, and focus are either building or draining your health.

Your health is a balance sheet, a running tally of assets and liabilities. Every choice you make either adds to your vitality or subtracts from it. Very simply, assets are the behaviors that build vitality. Liabilities are the factors that drain it.

Think of this exercise like sitting down with a financial planner. What does the planner do? They help you take inventory. They show you your assets and liabilities. And most importantly, they help you see where you are most exposed, where risks could compound if left unaddressed. Life equity works the same way.

Virtue compounds just like interest. Every daily decision adds or subtracts from your life's equity. Unlike money, vitality cannot be borrowed or bought. It must be earned through consistent alignment with your highest values.

Franklin never achieved moral perfection, and neither will you. But in pursuing it, he became one of the most disciplined and influential men in history. The pursuit itself transformed him.

Use the scoring system below to calculate your Vitality Balance and determine areas for improvement. A higher score reflects better metabolic health and vitality. The factors assessed are not just one-time events. They carry compounding liability. The longer they go unchecked, the more they eat away at your body's reserves. On the other side of the coin, the earlier you address them, the better your return. Imagine the value for your children and grandchildren.

Assets: Positive Contributions to Vitality

Rate each item from 0 (never) to 10 (daily) based on how consistently you've engaged in or experienced this behavior over the past thirty days.

Note: Be honest, this assessment is designed to guide improvement, not judge.

Asset: *Rate the positive health behaviors you practice.*	*Score 0–10*
I eat a nutrient-dense, whole-food diet (minimal sugar, processed food, seed oils).	
I drink at least half my body weight in ounces of clean, filtered water daily.	
I stop eating at least two hours before bed.	
I take high-quality supplements that meet my personal nutrient needs.	
I intentionally move my body daily for at least twenty minutes (walking, training, stretching, etc.).	
I engage in resistance training at least twice per week.	
I practice deep, diaphragmatic breathing or breath-focused exercises.	
I maintained seven to eight hours of quality, uninterrupted sleep each night.	
I maintain a consistent sleep/wake rhythm.	
I include greens, fiber, or gut-supportive foods regularly.	
I start my day with peace-building practices (e.g., prayer, Scripture, stillness).	
I practice daily gratitude or affirmations to shape thought patterns.	
I intentionally limit time with negative people or environments that drain me.	
I get adjusted regularly by a principled, neurologically focused chiropractor.	
I engage in postural and spinal alignment training exercises daily.	
I only use paraben and fragrance-free cosmetics, deodorants, and personal care products.	
I spent at least thirty minutes outside in the sunlight.	

Asset: *Rate the positive health behaviors you practice.*	*Score 0–10*
I avoid artificial flavors, food dyes, and additives in my food and beverages.	
I minimize blue light and screen exposure before bed (or use blue light blockers).	
I take intentional breaks from screens or technology throughout the day to reset my focus and energy.	

Liabilities: Drains on Vitality

Rate each item from 0 (never) to 10 (daily) based on how consistently you've engaged in or experienced this behavior over the past thirty days.

*   *Note: Be honest—this assessment is designed to guide improvement, not judge.**

Liabilities: *Rate the behaviors or exposures that negatively impact your vitality*	*Score 0–10*
I consumed processed or sugary foods/drinks.	
I skipped movement or was mostly sedentary. *(10 = No exercise; 0 = Regular, intentional physical activity.)*	
I experienced high stress without intentional practices to promote peace.	
When I ate beef, it was conventional beef (grain-fed and often exposed to antibiotics or hormones).	
When I ate chicken or eggs, it was conventional chicken (caged and often exposed to antibiotics or hormones).	
I relied on fast food or highly processed convenience foods.	
I slept on my stomach.	
I consumed alcohol, smoked, or used nicotine-based products.	
I spent more than two hours on screens without breaks, blue light protection, or movement.	
I consumed sugary drinks (soda, sweetened coffee/tea, energy drinks).	
I spent little to no time outdoors or in sunlight.	
I rely on medications, whether over the counter or prescriptive, for symptom management (excluding essential treatments for certain conditions).	

(Continued on next page)

Liabilities: Rate the behaviors or exposures that negatively impact your vitality	Score 0–10
I rely heavily on convenience foods.	
I use artificial sweeteners or consume foods or drinks labeled as "low-fat" or "diet."	
I regularly get annual vaccinations (in the last year).	
I stay up past 11 p.m. at least several nights per week.	
I use screens within one hour of bedtime without blue light protection.	
I stay in emotionally draining environments without boundaries.	
I eat or snack late at night (within one hour of bedtime).	
I eat distracted, while working, driving, or scrolling, rather than present and focused.	

Calculate Your Vitality Balance
1. *Add up your total score for the "Assets" section.*
2. *Add up your total score for the "Liabilities" section.*
3. *Subtract your Liabilities Total from your Assets Total:*
*Compare your score to the grading scale below

Vitality Grading Scale

Score Range	Category	Interpretation
+150 to +200	**Optimal Vitality**	You're living in alignment with your design. Your nervous system is regulated, your resilience is high, and you're actively restoring health. Maintain this standard.
+90 to +149	**Living Vital**	A strong foundation. You've built consistency, but some liabilities still drain your system. Refine and level up.
+30 to +89	**Vulnerable**	You're headed in the right direction, but imbalance is building. Strengthen your weakest areas before symptoms escalate.

Score Range	Category	Interpretation
0 to +29	**High Risk**	Your body is stuck in defense mode. You're doing some things right, but the system is under pressure. It's time to shift, hard.
Below 0	**Critical**	Your nervous system is overwhelmed. You're surviving, not thriving. Immediate, decisive action is needed to restore function and reclaim vitality.

Example Calculation

Assets (Positive Contributions to Vitality)

Asset Behavior	Score
Nutrient-dense meals	8
Hydration	9
Eating 2+ hours before bed	5
High-quality supplementation	7
Daily movement (20+ min)	6
Resistance training (2x/week)	4
Deep, diaphragmatic breathing	5
Seven to eight hours of quality sleep	8
Consistent sleep/wake rhythm	6
Fiber, greens, gut support	9
Morning peace practices (prayer, etc.)	7
Gratitude or affirmations	5
Limiting toxic relationships	6
Regular chiropractic adjustments	10
Alignment training exercises	3
Nontoxic personal care products	4
30+ min sunlight exposure	7
Avoiding artificial additives/dyes	6
Blue light protection before bed	5
Intentional tech breaks	4

Assets Total: 140

Liabilities (Drains on Vitality)

Liability Behavior	Score
Processed/sugary food intake	6
Sedentary behavior	4
Unmanaged stress	7
Conventional beef consumption	5
Conventional chicken/eggs	6
Fast food	3
Stomach sleeping	6
Alcohol/smoking/nicotine	2
Excessive screen time without breaks	6
Sugary beverages	3
Little to no outdoor time	2
Overreliance on meds for symptoms	8
Frequent convenience foods	4
Artificial sweeteners/diet foods	5
Routine vaccinations in past year	10
Staying up past 11 p.m.	6
No blue light protection at night	6
Emotionally toxic relationships	6
Eating while distracted (e.g., scrolling, driving)	7
Late-night snacking	5

Liabilities Total: 113

Category	Score
Assets Total	140
Liabilities Total	113
Vitality Balance (Assets minus Liabilities)	+27
Category	**High Risk**

No matter where you scored on the Vitality Balance Sheet, the most important thing is that you were honest. This isn't about getting a perfect score, it's about getting a clear score. Because clarity is power. You can't build real vitality on wishful thinking. You can't get where you want to go by lying to yourself about where you are. If you scored lower than you hoped, that's not failure, that's feedback. And feedback is what gives you the leverage to change. Most people stay stuck because they believe their current situation permanently defines them or they simply haven't been given the opportunity to do a quality assessment. But the ones who transform their health, their energy, and their life? They start by owning exactly where they stand and knowing that change is possible.

Vitality isn't about being perfect. It's about being consistent. What you do occasionally doesn't define your health, what you do repeatedly does. If you eat clean for a week and then binge on junk for two, that's your real pattern. If you exercise hard for a few days but then sit for weeks, that's your reality. But here's the good news: the opposite is also true. If you consistently make even small, strategic improvements, those habits compound into something powerful. Vitality isn't built in a day, it's built in your daily choices. And now that you have an honest assessment of where you are, you have the opportunity to start making those choices with real intention.

This chapter is your turning point. The next layer isn't just learning about health, it's experiencing it. Each of the next chapters will guide you through the practical application of the seven virtues, showing you exactly how to integrate these principles into your daily life.

Vitality isn't a mystery. It's the result of daily decisions. Start with the Vitality Balance Sheet, then pick the low-hanging fruit: eliminate what's draining you or double down where you're weakest. Small, consistent wins create momentum, and momentum rewires everything.

Vitality in Action: Applying the Vitality Balance Sheet

Now that you've assessed where you are, it's time to put that clarity to work. The Vitality Balance Sheet is a road map. You now have a clear picture of your health assets (the habits that are working for you) and your health liabilities (the patterns that are holding you back). The next step is to take strategic action, not by overhauling everything at once, but by making consistent, focused improvements in the areas that matter most.

1. Double Down on Your Assets

Identify one high-impact asset that's easy to implement and commit to making it a daily habit for the next thirty days. Example: If you're not staying hydrated, start drinking half your body weight in ounces of water daily. Pair it with a trigger, like drinking a glass of water first thing in the morning.

Your strengths are your foundation. Instead of only focusing on what's wrong, amplify what's already working. The fastest way to build momentum is to reinforce a habit that supports your vitality. By doubling down on what's working, you're reinforcing behaviors that naturally crowd out bad habits and make the next step easier.

2. Neutralize One Liability That's Draining You Most

Look at your liabilities and pick one behavior that's dragging your vitality down the most. Commit to replacing it with a positive behavior for the next week. Example: If late-night eating is your struggle, replace it with an evening routine like herbal tea, stretching, or journaling.

Every liability is costing you vitality, but some are more damaging than others. If you try to fix everything at once, you'll fail. Instead, pick the one habit that's draining you the most and start there.

3. Stack Wins and Expand

After thirty days, stack another habit. Keep using the Vitality Balance Sheet to track your progress and adjust. One good habit isn't enough, but it's the first domino. Once you've locked in a new positive behavior, build on it. This is how you create sustainable vitality that compounds over time. Example: If you started with hydration, add a movement goal, like walking five thousand steps daily or stretching every morning.

Momentum is your greatest tool. The more assets you build, the stronger your foundation becomes. Stay consistent, stay adaptable, and keep stacking wins. This isn't about chasing perfection, it's about making vitality your default.

The Seven Virtues are more than a philosophy. They give you a foundation with direction. When you put them into action, they will help you untangle health issues, remove interference, and move toward vitality with clarity.

They don't add more to your plate. They shift how you see, think, and choose. They become a guide for how you live. That's where we go next.

We begin with the virtue of Mental Fortitude, because what you believe sets the direction for everything that follows. That's why it's essential to rewire the mind. If your thoughts are shaped by fear, control, or resignation, your choices will reflect that. But the moment you create new mental pathways, you reclaim your ability to heal, to flourish, and to live with vitality.

CHAPTER 16

Rewire the Mind

For though we walk in the flesh, we are not waging war according to the flesh. For the weapons of our warfare are not of the flesh but have divine power to destroy strongholds. We destroy arguments and every lofty opinion raised against the knowledge of God, and take every thought captive to obey Christ.

—2 Corinthians 10:3–5 (ESV)

The Virtue of Mental Fortitude

Health freedom requires us to return to natural order. But only when we see differently will we begin to live differently.

This might be the most important chapter in the book. Shifting from the medical model to a life of vitality requires rewiring the mind. Without it, you'll keep defaulting to the same reference points of symptom treatment, expert dependency, and fear-based decisions.

I say this with confidence because the systems we rely on, whether insurance, education, food policy, or even health advice from trusted institutions, are all built on allopathic assumptions. Unless you have already done the deep work to rewire your thinking, the old paradigm will keep pulling you back.

To reclaim your health, you'll have to step off Medicine's playing field and onto the field of vitality. The two don't share the same map. One views the body as broken and dangerous. The other sees it as intelligent, expressive, responsive, and designed to heal.

A Note from Leah

I can't think of a better application of the significance and practice of rewiring your thoughts than pregnancy and birth. After a decade-long fertility journey and a second-trimester loss in my late thirties, I chose differently with the surprise conception of my rainbow baby, MJ. Early on, I resolved that any provider who brought fear into the journey would not walk it with me.

Bringing MJ earthside tested my faith in every way. And God showed up.

Every pregnancy presents a fork in the road: fear or faith. From the time of conception, women step into a model of care that recasts pregnancy as a dangerous condition to manage, tracked by labs, ultrasounds, and constant surveillance. But when we pause to reflect on the brilliance of two cells multiplying into trillions, forming a beating heart and a whole new life, it becomes clear: **Medicine has nothing to add to this miracle.**

Modern maternity care layers pregnancy with fear. Interventions are framed as "necessary," but no intervention is without consequence.

- **Inductions**, often presented as routine, can lead to fetal distress and increased risk of C-section.
- **Epidurals** cross the placenta and can lead to hypoxic effects in the baby.
- **Ultrasounds** expose the baby to heat and high-frequency sound that may disrupt fetal development and restrict uterine growth. Many of the conditions flagged by ultrasound resolve on their own. The fear they induce does not.
- **Doppler waves** generate heat and mechanical vibrations in tissues and carry risks for fetal development.
- **C-sections** are sometimes lifesaving, but frequently overused, leading to higher risks for both mom and baby—including infection, hemorrhage, respiratory issues in newborns, and long-term effects on the infant microbiome and immune development.

Pregnancy and birth are sacred biological processes. It is an unmatched opportunity to cocreate *with* God. To trust Him instead of man's knowledge with what is most precious. The fear-based patterns accepted during pregnancy as normal do not disappear when the baby arrives. They echo into infancy, fueling postpartum anxiety and depression at unprecedented rates. Here are a few of the shifts I experienced to exit the matrix of fear:

Medical Mindset	Vitality Mindset
Measure and test everything *looking for problems* (from due dates to size, dilation, contractions, and hours of labor) → cascade of interventions	Trust the process and *expect things to go well* → little to zero intervention *Testing only happens if a sign or symptom warns of a concern and the outcome of the test will impact decision-making
Avoid pain; plan the birth	Belief that the body is doing the right thing at the right time; support the natural process
Hyperfocus on baby's position	Optimize mom's movement and alignment and baby will be in the perfect position at the perfect time

Choosing faith over fear rewires your pregnancy, reshapes your motherhood, and redefines your child's future.

Simply adding new habits on top of an old belief system is futile. You have to retrain the way you think. You have to rewire your mind. Otherwise, the next time you come to a point of decision, you will be stuck in old solutions. Medicine has governed America's health and healthcare for five generations with the "old solutions" as the only option. But it's time for families to take back the driver's seat. That means rejecting the paradigm that treats every symptom as a tragedy and every diagnosis as a new identity. That mindset, rooted in victimhood and toxic empathy, is incompatible with healing and leads to bondage.

Pain is not always a problem to eliminate. Most often, it's a signal. Suffering can be a starting point on a journey, not a life sentence. Only when we learn to see differently will we begin to live differently. And living differently changes your brain.

Your brain is not fixed. It's rewiring every second, based on what you think, believe, repeat, and dwell on. We discussed neuroplasticity in depth in part 2, and while science gets the credit for naming it, Scripture has long offered the same insight by telling us to "take every thought captive."

Your brain is designed to be shaped by experience. You either take your thoughts captive and shape your experiences, or your experiences (especially trauma) will shape you. And they won't ask permission. There is a war for your mind, and most people are losing by default because they don't even know they're under attack and thus are not engaging in the battle.

If you believe there are forces of good and evil in this world, then it would follow that the enemy's primary strategy is deception. If you believe a lie and repeat it long enough, the enemy doesn't need chains. You'll live in a cage of your own making. This stands in stark contrast to the ownership required for vitality. It's captivity.

That's how strongholds are built. Thought by thought . . . over time.

How to Take Every Thought Captive

Taking thoughts captive isn't a metaphor. It's a spiritual *and* neurological strategy.

Here's how to do it in real time:

1. **Notice the thought and name it.**

   Catch tormenting, unproductive, or dark thoughts before they go deeper or become a spiral. Your best indicator or trigger to notice the thought is often physical cues such as your chest tightening or mind racing or it might be emotional with a sudden sense of feeling trapped or unsettled or a sense of dread.

   What is this thought *actually* saying? If your thought is a frazzled, "I have too much to do today." the deeper belief might actually be, "I'm not enough." or "I can't handle this." Say it plainly. Call it out.

2. **Test it.**

   Hold it up to biblical virtue. Is it noble, pure, lovely, admirable, just, praiseworthy, honorable (Philippians 4:8)?

   If not, it's not true. Period.

3. Speak back.

Use truth to dismantle the lie. Out loud. Boldly. God does not want you to be fearful or insecure. His power is at work in you.

God has not given me a spirit of fear but of power, love, and a sound mind. 2 Timothy 1:7 (NKJV)

This is not affirmation or simply self-help. This is spiritual warfare. Notice that you are inserting a true, life-giving thought in its place. Don't just reject lies, speak truth.

Every time you do this, you forge new neural pathways. You're not just believing differently. You're becoming transformed by the renewing of your mind.

Do not be conformed to this world, but be transformed by the renewal of your mind, that by testing you may discern what is the will of God, what is good and acceptable and perfect.

—(Romans 12:2 ESV)

This verse captures the entire chapter in one punch, your transformation begins in the mind, but not by passively avoiding lies. By renewing your mind daily, you build mental resilience. You fortify.

Build a Fortified Mind

To fortify something means to strengthen it against attack, to surround it with defenses that hold firm when pressure mounts. In ancient times, cities were fortified with walls, towers, and gates. They were built to protect what mattered most inside.

Your mind is no different. If it's not fortified, the body is vulnerable. The Greek word for "fortress" "ochyrōma" (ὀχύρωμα) is the same word Paul, in the Bible, used for *strongholds*. But here's the twist: strongholds can be defensive or destructive.

Building a fortified mind means building defensive strongholds: protection, peace, discernment. Lies and repeated deception build destructive strongholds: fear, anxiety, hopelessness.

Perhaps this is why the Bible instructs us to "take every thought captive" (2 Corinthians 10:5).

The word for *captive* "aichmalōtizō" (αἰχμαλωτίζω) means to take by spearpoint. It's active, violent, intentional. You don't entertain thoughts. You test and interrogate them. You don't let them "pass through." You arrest them.

To rewire the brain is to fortify the mind. To fortify the mind is to live with mental sovereignty, where you decide what enters, what stays, and what gets replaced. So how do you do that? You don't just think harder or pray once and hope it sticks. You don't wish it into existence. You train for it.

Here are six practices to help you build a fortified mindset by being "transformed by the renewal of your mind."

1. Start Your Day on Purpose

How you begin your day decides who gets the first voice in your life. Before emails, headlines, or alerts dictate your mind, anchor in truth. Some simple alliterations to help you start the day with sound, sober-mindedness:

- Scripture before screen
- Prayer before pressure
- Breath before busyness
- Gratitude before grind

Start the Day on Purpose

Write it down:

Create your Morning Grounding Routine. What will you do in the first ten minutes to fortify your mind?

Options to choose from:

- Scripture reading
- Breathwork (alignment breath trio)
- Sunwalking
- Gratitude
- Prayer or worship

Circle two to three practices to start tomorrow

---

2. Practice Peace Management

Whatever you think about grows. Whatever you focus on expands. So why are we obsessed with *managing stress*? Do you really want to manage your stress? Keep it organized, wear it like a badge, let it shape your nervous system?

Stop treating stress like it's something to avoid or villainize. Stress is an inevitable part of life. You'll stress yourself out trying to avoid it. Instead, focus on building resilience. Start managing peace like it's a cherished asset (because it is).

And that's exactly why peace must be built, and often fought for. This happens by active pursuit not by simply being free spirited. *Turn away from evil and do good; seek peace and pursue it.* (Psalm 34:14). The word *peace* is shalom, which means wholeness, completeness, nothing is missing, not to be confused with passivity or softness. It's the full restoration of order in your mind, your body, your relationships, and your spirit. But peace doesn't come by avoiding conflict. It comes by confronting what is out of order.

Peace is also not the absence of struggle, it's the result of setting things right. Throughout many historical texts, shalom comes after repentance, battle, truth, and justice restored. Sometimes peace means confronting lies and breaking sin patterns.

> *Put on the full armor of God, so that when the day of evil comes, you may be able to stand your ground . . . with the readiness that comes from the gospel of peace.*
>
> —(Ephesians 6:13;15)

Here's how to start training for it daily:

- Confront and cut off anything in your life that creates disconnect from God
- Take every thought captive
- Dismantle old patterns that keep you stuck
- Reject internal chaos and external distractions

It will serve you well to abandon the futile practice of either avoiding or managing stress. Instead train your mind to dwell in peace and actively pursue shalom. Because that kind of peace is a weapon that wins the battle of the mind.

Interrupt the Thought Loop
Write it down:

Next time fear, anxiety creeps in, pause and ask:

- Is this true?
- Is this useful?
- Does it hold up to Biblical virtue?

Then replace the thought with truth. Write your go-to Scripture or truth here:

_____

_____

_____

3. Shape Your Environment

You can't rewire your brain while living in a constant state of mental assault. Your environment either fortifies your mind or fractures it.

Fortify your environment by:

- Filtering the news
- Pruning your social feeds (or eliminating altogether)
- Setting firm boundaries around draining people

Call it guarding your gates. Not everything or everyone gets access.

Guard the Gates
Write it down:

What drains you daily that you've allowed through your gates? Where are the leaks in your mental environment?

List three boundaries you need to set, or reset.

1. _____
2. _____
3. _____

4. Wire Your Brain for Gratitude

Building the muscle of gratitude is a winning strategy for success in relationships, in reaching your goals, and in your health. Epigenetics shows that your cells literally strengthen in response to gratitude. Whenever you remove a thought, the reason we replace it intentionally is because a void will be filled. Your brain is wired to spot threats for mere survival. So without intentional practice, you'll default to what's missing, broken, or frustrating. But just thirty seconds of real, spoken gratitude can activate your parasympathetic nervous system and bring restoration to your body.

In our family, we practice "three things you're thankful for" at night during devotional time. We started this practice to specifically benefit one family member that was earning the nickname Eeyore. At first, it wasn't always easy. But it shifts the atmosphere within each family member and within the home, every single time. Gratitude doesn't just change your mood. It reshapes your mind.

Anchor with Gratitude
Write it down:

List three specific things you're grateful for today. Speak them out loud. *Pro tip: Do this for ten straight days and track how your sleep or emotional state changes by day seven.*

1. _____
2. _____
3. _____

5. Establish a Strong Room

You're not meant to do this alone. Jim Rohn said you are the average of the five people you spend the most time with. Basically, your mom was right when she had an opinion about your friends and beat into your head that you are who you hang out with.

One of my mentors called it your strong room: the circle of people you intentionally choose as an adult, who reflect the values you want to grow into. These are your anchors and even though they may never be in the same room together, they make up your proverbial strong room. When you are assessing your current strong room or building it going forward, take a look at who espouses the values you want to emulate in each of the following categories. A person might fill multiple of these categories, and they might not:

1. Spiritual and emotional
2. Financial and business
3. Family and spouse
4. Fitness and nutrition

You don't need more opinions. You need anchors.

Write it down:
Now list the five people you want influencing your growth.
1. _____
2. _____
3. _____
4. _____
5. _____

Where do you need to shift access or pursue new alignment?
_____
_____

CHAPTER 17

Sleep, Rest, and Recovery

Sleep is the single most effective thing we can do to reset our brain and body health each day.

—Matthew Walker, *Why We Sleep*

The Virtue of Rest

I used to believe that if you just cleaned up your food, moved your body, and got your stress under control, sleep would take care of itself. I don't believe that anymore.

Sleep is the biological foundation everything else depends on. If you weaken sleep, your nervous system stays stuck in survival mode. You can eat clean, take the best supplements, and follow a flawless workout plan but if you're not sleeping, you're trying to run a high-performance engine on dirty fuel. When sleep is shallow or sporadic, no part of your biology escapes the consequences.

- **Your nervous system stays stuck in sympathetic dominance.** This keeps your body inflamed, tense, and reactive.
- **Hormones misfire.** Cortisol, melatonin, growth hormone, insulin, and leptin all depend on sleep to sync their cycles.
- **Your brain never detoxes.** The glymphatic system, the brain's waste removal system, only flushes at night. That's when it clears out beta-amyloid, the same plaque linked to Alzheimer's.
- **Your immune system weakens.** Without deep sleep, natural killer cells plummet and inflammation rises. After just one night

204

of sleep restricted to four hours, natural killer (NK) cell activity drops to 72 percent of baseline, weakening your first line of immune defense.[1]

- **Your cravings skyrocket.** Disrupted sleep deregulates leptin and ghrelin, tipping hunger and satiety out of balance.

If that wasn't enough, there are some other shocking statistics. Men who sleep five hours or less have significantly smaller testicles than those who sleep seven or more.[2] Memory recall drops by 40 percent in the sleep-deprived.[3] And just one week of sleeping six hours a night alters the expression of over 700 genes, many of them tied to immune dysfunction and cancer.[4]

Sleep and Metabolism: The Leptin-Ghrelin Disruption

If you're sleeping less than six hours a night and can't seem to get control of your appetite, it's not just a willpower issue, it becomes hormonal.

Dr. Eve Van Cauter out of the University of Chicago ran a series of studies that changed everything we thought we knew about sleep and metabolism.

In one study, she took two groups of healthy participants and gave them the same food and physical activity. The only difference? One group had 8.5 hours of sleep per night, and the other had just four to five hours.

By the fifth night, the short-sleep group had significantly lower levels of leptin (the "I'm full" hormone) and higher levels of ghrelin (the "I'm hungry" hormone). They weren't moving their bodies more. They weren't eating less. And yet their hunger signals were out of control.[5]

Bottom line: less sleep made them ravenous. Their cravings went up, especially for processed carbs and sugar. And their ability to feel satisfied? Gone.

In a follow-up study with the same sleep conditions, Van Cauter's team gave participants free access to food. They meticulously counted the calories consumed by both groups. The result? The sleep-deprived group ate an average of three hundred more calories per day. That adds up to more than one thousand extra calories over just five days.[6]

Now do the math: three hundred extra calories per day over the course of a year = thirty-one pounds of potential weight gain. All from disrupted sleep and a hijacked hormonal feedback loop. Sleep loss doesn't just make you tired. It makes you metabolically vulnerable.

Nutrients Needed for Sleep

When you sleep, your body gets out of defense mode and into regulation. Every system begins to heal when your body surrenders to deep, consistent sleep. And beyond the rhythms and hormones, sleep quality also depends on whether your body has the right raw materials.

If you're depleted in magnesium, glycine, GABA, or L-theanine, your body may struggle to downshift. These nutrients are needed for relaxing the nervous system, lowering cortisol, and allowing melatonin to rise. If serotonin is low, your brain won't convert enough into melatonin, and without enough 5-HTP, that conversion stalls.

Nutrient deficiency can hijack your ability to sleep even if your habits are perfect. That's why we don't treat supplementation as optional when rebuilding that rhythm. Replenish depleted nutrients, remove the barriers that interfere with deep sleep and watch your brain begin to reset.

The Seven-Point Sleep Audit
Is Sleep Your Asset or Your Liability?
Put a ✓ next to every statement that's consistently true for you:

- I fall asleep within fifteen to thirty minutes most nights
- I sleep seven to nine hours without frequent wakeups
- I wake up without needing an alarm clock
- I feel alert and focused during the day
- I don't need caffeine or sugar to survive the morning
- I limit screens at least sixty minutes before bed
- I get sunlight within thirty minutes of waking

Results:
- **Six to seven checks:** Rhythm is solid. Fine-tune and protect it.
- **Fourt to five checks:** On the edge, time to reinforce better habits.
- **Three or fewer:** Sleep is a liability. Rewire it now.

Barriers That Wreck Sleep

These habits sabotage your sleep and recovery. Put a ✓ next to every barrier that's true for you:

- Screens before bed (especially in bed)
- Falling asleep with the TV on
- Alcohol in the evening (destroys REM)
- High-intensity workouts late in the day
- Heavy carbs or sugar after dinner

Reset Sleep: Practical Rewire Actions

If you aren't getting consistent, 7+ hours of sleep or you scored three or fewer in the Seven-Point Sleep Audit, the below isn't a list of suggestions. These are nonnegotiables if you want to regulate your nervous system and restore rhythm.

1. **Stop eating two to three hours before bed:** Food raises insulin and cortisol. That delays melatonin and blocks deep sleep.
2. **Protect your light environment after sunset:** Blue light from screens tells your brain it's daytime. Use blue-light blockers, dim lights, and install *f.lux* on your devices.
3. **Anchor your wake-up time:** Your circadian rhythm locks on to your wake-up time. Pick one and stick to it, even on weekends.
4. **Get sunlight within thirty minutes of waking:** Morning light raises cortisol at the right time and triggers melatonin release twelve to fourteen hours later.
5. **Build a wind-down routine:** Trade screen-scrolling for breathwork, prayer, stretching, or journaling. These tell your brain it's time to switch off.
6. **Supplement if needed:** To address nutrient depletion or deficiencies, use:
   - BioAvail Magnesium (by Vitality Metabolics)—200–400 mg of magnesium glycinate before bed

- Reset PM (by Vitality Metabolics)—includes GABA, L-theanine, 5-HTP
- Glycine or tart cherry extract for additional support

Write It Down: Your Next Sleep Step
What's one thing you're ready to change starting *tonight*?
- Move your phone out of the bedroom?
- Ditch late-night snacks?
- Turn screens off an hour earlier?

Write it down. Make it real.
I will _____in order to protect my sleep rhythm.
Post it somewhere you'll see it before bed.

Vitality in Action: Reset Sleep Protocol
Tonight:
- Eat dinner three hours before bed
- Shut down screens sixty minutes before sleep
- Try Navy SEAL Breath
- Take BioAvail Magnesium (200–400 mg)
- Sleep in a dark, cool room, phone out of reach

Tomorrow Morning:
- Get outside within thirty minutes of waking
- Anchor your wake time

Try it for five days. Notice the difference: clearer mind, steadier mood, deeper energy.

Let's not overcomplicate sleep. If you've already dialed in the basics like light, food, and rhythm and it's still off, it's time to look deeper. Often the missing piece isn't another sleep hack. It's how you move. That's what we're diving into next: movement as medicine.

CHAPTER 18

Repattern Movement and Breath

Effort in the wrong direction is not strength. It is mastery of the mistake.
—Stoic philosophy

The Virtue of Movement

If you're not moving well or regularly, your nervous system is stuck. And the solution isn't more repetitions or longer workouts, it's better signals. Movement tells your brain, *"I'm safe."* Breath tells it, *"I'm in control."* Together, they shift you out of survival and into regulation.

But it's not just *any* movement that matters, it's the *right* movement for your body's imbalances. That's where Alignment Training comes in.

What Is Alignment Training?

In practice, I've spent years witnessing the struggles that people face with poor posture, weak core engagement, and chronically imbalanced muscles. In the past, I would often prescribe exercises that required thirty minutes twice per day to be effective.

But despite the best intentions, many of my practice members found it difficult to stay consistent. The exercises were too time-consuming, and they weren't effectively addressing two of the major problems: muscle imbalances and lack of core engagement. This made the goal of improving spinal alignment, already a challenging task, even harder. This frustration led me to create Alignment Training.

Alignment Training is a nervous system-based movement system that retrains posture, breath, and muscle balance. Although I created a very convenient way for you to integrate Alignment Training into your daily routine, you don't necessarily have to use my program. This chapter will teach you how to integrate breath, posture, and neurological-based movements, all of which are the foundation of Alignment Training. It's not about how hard you train. It's about how intelligently you move.

The Core of Alignment Training

- You train based on your body's unique alignment pattern (we'll walk through each in a moment).
- You use corrective movements to stabilize weak areas and downshift overactive ones.
- You reconnect breathing, posture, and nervous system balance, instead of chasing workouts that create more tension or inflammation.
- Most people exercise on top of dysfunction. Alignment Training corrects the dysfunction first and then moves to subsequent phases of retraining posture and neurology.

Why It Works

- **Movement** = Safety Signal
  Rhythmic, intentional motion tells your brain, *"I'm not under threat."*
- **Breath** = Regulation Lever
  The way you breathe directly affects vagal tone, emotional state, and functional movement patterns.
- **Posture** = Nervous System Feedback
  Slouched posture feeds collapse. Upright alignment sends power and presence back into your system.

Your Alignment Type: The Seven Patterns

Most people are stuck in movement patterns shaped by years of sitting, stress, and survival. These patterns show up in your posture, breathing, strength imbalances, and even your energy levels.

Alignment Training starts by identifying your default pattern, then retrains your body with movements that restore balance, stability, and nervous system flow. So, which one are you? Below are the seven most common Alignment Types. See if you can identify which one is you.

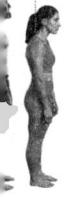

1. **Closed Off**
   - Distinguishing feature: excessive curvature in the upper back (thoracic hyperkyphosis)
   - Typical signs: forward head, rounded shoulders, collapsed chest
   - Nervous system state: self-protective, sometimes withdrawn
   - Training focus: open the chest, strengthen postural muscles, restore extension

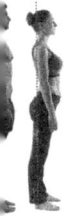

2. **Gymnast**
   - Distinguishing feature: excessive curvature in the lower back (lumbar hyperlordosis)
   - Typical signs: arched back, flared ribs, tight hip flexors
   - Nervous system state: Performance-driven, often sympathetically dominant
   - Training focus: downregulate lumbar extension, strengthen core and glutes

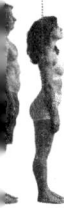

3. **Duck**
   - Distinguishing feature: flat upper back and excessive lower back curve
   - Typical signs: neck pushed forward, hips arched back, anterior pelvic tilt
   - Nervous system state: pulled into forward drive, overcompensating
   - Training focus: recenter spine, reset breath, retrain core-pelvis connection

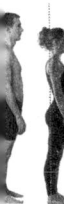

4. **Curvy**
   - Distinguishing feature: excessive curvature in both upper and lower spine

- Typical signs: rounded upper back and arched low back, compression in midsection
- Nervous system state: tense, overactive, hyperreactive
- Training focus: expand posture, stabilize deep core, reduce global tension

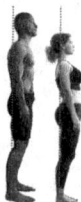

5. Flatback
- Distinguishing feature: loss of natural curvature in lower back
- Typical signs: tucked pelvis, tight hamstrings, rigid torso
- Nervous system state: guarded, bracing, energy-conserving
- Training focus: restore lumbar curve, open hips, reestablish spinal rhythm

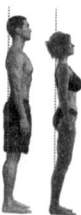

6. Ruler
- Distinguishing feature: loss of curvature in both upper and lower spine
- Typical signs: straight posture, but rigid and stiff; no natural flow
- Nervous system state: over-controlled, locked down
- Training focus: restore spinal curves, reintegrate breath and fluid motion

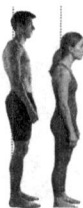

7. Tech
- Distinguishing feature: upper spine overly curved and lower spine flattened
- Typical signs: text-neck posture, flat hips, rib depression
- Nervous system state: overstimulated and collapsed
- Training focus: rebuild upper back strength, support lower spine, restore rib cage dynamics

Go to fxalign.com /reclaimvitality to take the Alignment Quiz to find your pattern and start retraining your posture from the inside system out.

These patterns aren't cosmetic. They're neurological. They shape how you breathe, digest, move, and think. Left uncorrected, each one creates predictable stress on the nervous system. And over time, that stress turns into symptoms.

Here's what happens when each pattern is ignored:

Alignment Type and the Cost of Ignoring It

Alignment Type	Long-Term Impact if Ignored
Tech	Shallow breathing, neck tension, brain fog, frequent headaches, restless sleep, forward collapse in posture
Closed Off	Slouched appearance, tight shoulders, poor oxygen flow, low confidence, tension headaches, emotional withdrawal
Curvy	Energy crashes, poor sleep, tight hips, trapped tension in the neck and low back, digestive issues, mood swings
Gymnast	Achy lower back, tight hip flexors, bloated stomach, trouble standing or sitting for long periods, poor posture awareness
Duck	Rib tightness, limited shoulder movement, anxiousness, bloating or sluggish digestion, low back tightness that doesn't go away
Flat Back	Stiff low back, lack of flexibility, poor balance, weak core feeling, sensitivity when sitting too long
Ruler	Rigid posture, difficulty relaxing, flat energy, anxiousness, off-balance feeling, poor tolerance to physical or emotional stress

What All Alignment Types Have in Common

No matter which pattern you fall into, you'll notice three key principles show up again and again:

1. **Focus on the Diaphragm and Deep Core**
   These are your foundation. When they're inactive, your body overcompensates, pulling tension into your low back, neck, and hips. Every pattern needs core restoration from the inside out.

2. **Incorporate Deep, Intentional Breathing**
   Shallow chest breathing reinforces stress and instability. Alignment Training uses breath to reset your nervous system and retrain your movement.

3. Avoid Movements That Reinforce Your Pattern

Most people keep strengthening the muscles that are already overactive. Without realizing it, they're training themselves *deeper into dysfunction*. That's why certain exercises, while popular, can actually make your alignment worse.

If you train the wrong pattern harder, you don't get stronger, you get more stuck.

Nervous System Balance > Muscle Balance

Most people try to fix imbalances by stretching or massaging what's tight and strengthening what's weak. Sounds logical, but it rarely works.

Why? Because the nervous system is still running the show. If a muscle is overactive, it's because your nervous system *wants* it that way. It's protecting you. Bracing. Compensating. Trying to create stability where it doesn't exist.

You can stretch that tight muscle all day. You can do hundreds of reps to "activate" the weak side. But if you haven't addressed the neurological imbalance underneath, it won't hold. You'll stay stuck. Progress will stall. Frustration sets in and most people quit right there.

It's not a discipline problem. It's a strategy problem. Once you know your Alignment Type, you stop guessing. You stop fighting your body. You move with precision, breathe with intention, and train your nervous system to stabilize from the inside out. That's when real change sticks.

Movement Is Medicine: Even a Walk Counts

Not all movement needs a mat or a program. One of the most neurologically restorative things you can do is also one of the simplest: walk. Especially outdoors. Especially in the morning.

Walking isn't just physical, it's primal. It recalibrates your vestibular system, regulates breathing, and activates the cross-crawl pattern that connects both hemispheres of your brain. Pair that with sunlight in your eyes and you've got a built-in circadian reset. That's nervous system regulation at its most ancient level.

Want a true reset? Wake up, walk toward the sun, breathe through your nose, and keep your gaze soft and wide. No phone. No distractions.

Just ten minutes of rhythmic, purposeful motion. This tells your body: *I'm safe. I'm stable. I'm awake.*

Stillness has its place. But you weren't made to be sedentary. You were made to move, and that movement doesn't need to be perfect. It just needs to be present.

Daily Reset: The Sunwalk Protocol

Want a daily rhythm to regulate your nervous system? Try this:

- Walk for at least ten minutes outdoors
- Face the morning sun for the first two to three minutes (no sunglasses). Gaze in the direction of the sun. Do not stare straight at the sun.
- Breathe through your nose in a slow, steady rhythm
- Keep your gaze soft and wide, avoid screens, focus on horizon or landscape

This combo resets your circadian rhythm, balances your visual system, and builds parasympathetic tone. No mat, no gear. Just you, the sun, and your breath.

Myth Buster: You Can't Foam Roll Your Way to Stability

Let's set the record straight:

- **Foam rolling** can reduce tension, but it doesn't retrain your nervous system.
- **Massage** feels great, but it doesn't fix faulty movement patterns.
- **Stretching tight muscles** without addressing alignment often reinforces the problem; it gives temporary relief while the system stays in dysfunction.

These tools aren't wrong, they're just incomplete.

Without restoring neurological balance, you're chasing symptoms, not correcting the pattern. If your body keeps reverting back after every massage, every "mobility day," or every perfect workout plan, it's not because you're broken. It's because you haven't addressed the system that controls it all. Train the nervous system. The muscles will follow.

The Eyes Lead the Spine

If the nervous system is the operating system of your body, then your eyes are the cursor. Where your eyes go, your head follows. Where your head goes, your spine follows. And where your spine goes, the rest of your body compensates.

Most people think poor posture starts in the shoulders or hips, but it often starts upstream, in the eyes. Staring down at screens. Locked into one focal distance all day. Overusing peripheral vision while underusing gaze stability. That's because your vestibular system (inner ear) and visual system are deeply connected. If they're out of sync, your nervous system stays tense and reactive.

Poor gaze control increases neck tension, throws off balance (this is particularly problematic in patterns like the Tech, Closed Off, and Ruler). Eye tracking drills stimulate the cerebellum and help calm an overactive stress response. We use these eye tracking drills in the Alignment Training program to help retrain the muscles and rewire the nervous system.

A Simple Eye Tracking Drill (Try This Today)

1. Sit or stand in a neutral posture.
2. Hold both thumbs out in front of you at eye level.
3. Keep your head still and follow your thumb with just your eyes as you move it slowly left to right and switch thumbs.
4. Do ten slow passes.
5. Repeat up/down and diagonal, as long as you aren't dizzy.

This activates the part of your brain responsible for coordination, spatial awareness, and postural control, without a single rep or stretch. Because the nervous system is visual, and if you want to restore balance from the top down, you can't ignore the lens it sees through. That's why it's essential to incorporate eye tracking into your daily activities, especially if you are trying to retrain a known imbalance. Now imagine doing these types of eye exercises while also doing a banded exercise for your hip alignment or rounded shoulders. That's how we incorporate it into Alignment Training. When you combine this with deep-breathing exercises, you have the perfect recipe for transformation.

The Alignment Breathing Trio

Your breath is one of the fastest ways to regulate your nervous system, but not all breathing is created equal.

The Alignment Breathing Trio, briefly described in chapter 9, gives you three specific techniques, each designed to support a different state: focus, recovery, and postural reset. These aren't hacks. They're tools to retrain your brain-body connection, anytime, anywhere.

Use them strategically based on how you want to feel, and when you need to shift your state.

Navy SEAL Breath

This structured breath pattern is used by elite athletes and special forces. It sharpens focus and helps your nervous system stay calm under pressure by teaching your body to shift from fight-or-flight into a place of controlled strength.

How to Do It:

- Inhale through your nose for four seconds
- Hold for four seconds
- Exhale through your mouth for four seconds
- Hold for four seconds
- Repeat for three to five rounds

This is how you build mental toughness and shift into a composed, alert state under pressure. Great for mornings, mindset resets, or priming your system for movement.

Amen Breath

This calming breath activates your vagus nerve through resonance. The slow exhale paired with a low "Ahhh-men" helps downshift your nervous system and restore peace, physically and emotionally. It's the perfect way to close a session or reset from stress.

How to Do It:
- Inhale through your nose for five seconds
- Hold for two seconds
- Exhale slowly with a deep, low *"Ahhh-men"* for five to eight seconds
- Feel the vibration in your throat and chest
- Repeat for three to five rounds

This activates the vagus nerve, slows your heart rate, and drops you into deep recovery. Use it when you need to downshift, physically, emotionally, or spiritually.

Barrel Breath
Barrel breath trains your body to breathe with your diaphragm, not your chest. It strengthens your deep core muscles and restores the 360° expansion pattern that supports posture, spinal stability, and nervous system balance.

How to Do It:
- Inhale through your nose for four to six seconds
- Expand your ribs forward, sideways, and into your back (like a barrel)
- Exhale slowly through pursed lips for six to eight seconds
- Keep the breath smooth and steady
- Repeat for three to five rounds

**Optional: Wrap a band or hands around your ribs to feel the 360° expansion

This trains your diaphragm, deep core, and postural system together. Over time, it rewires your breath and improves spinal stability without even thinking about it.

Putting It All Together: How to Do Alignment Training

I've already done the heavy lifting for you. The full Alignment Training program gives you the exact exercises to do, day by day, with zero guess-work. It's a no-think system that adapts as your body changes. But I also believe you deserve to understand the process, not just follow it.

So in this section, I'm giving you the recipe. You'll learn the core structure behind Alignment Training, how to reset your breath, target what's overactive, and retrain the reflexes your nervous system depends on. You can use this framework to create your own pattern-specific reset, anytime.

Simple. Strategic. Repeatable. This is how you start training your nervous system from the inside out.

Alignment Training Is Simple by Design:

- **One daily breath reset** (choose from the Alignment Breathing Trio)
- **Four to five targeted exercises** that release what's overactive and activate what's underperforming
- **Incorporate eye tracking** whenever possible to retrain visual reflexes and coordination

Example: Tech Pattern Reset (see fxalign.com/reclaimvitality for video)
Barrel Breath
Breath-based core activation
Cervical Retract and Reach
- Sit or stand tall
- Gently tuck chin to create a "double chin"
- Reach both arms forward while keeping spine tall
- Activate deep neck flexors and upper back

Scapular Protraction in High Plank
- Start in a strong plank: hands under shoulders, hips level
- Press the chest away from the floor by spreading the shoulder blades apart

- Hold briefly, then let chest drop to squeeze shoulder blades together
- Maintain head alignment and full core engagement

Seated Leg Lift
- Sit tall, legs straight in front of you
- Place a small object (foam block, towel, etc.) under one leg
- Brace your core and lift one leg slowly without leaning back
- Alternate sides. Goal: activate hip flexors without spinal compensation

Cervical Retract and Reach with Eye Tracking
- Begin in a hands-and-knees position
- Tuck chin, engage deep neck flexors
- Reach one arm forward, spine steady
- Move your eyes side to side without moving your head
- Progression: Hover knees in bear crawl position, add wider reach

Alignment Training is one of your tools to rewire from the inside out. But accuracy and consistency are paramount.

Why Most People Never Change and How to Beat the Pattern

The biggest challenge with any new routine is staying consistent. What do most people do? The same three stretches or "go-to" drills, day after day, until the brain tunes it out and the results flatline. That's why I created the Alignment Training program.

It takes out the guesswork. Every movement is built for your pattern. The flow changes on a regular basis. The system is intentional. All you have to do is show up.

Whether you're in pain, stuck in stress mode, or just tired of work-outs that aren't for you, this is your nervous system reset. No equipment. No guesswork. Just the right input, every day. Start training with intention.

Want a Done-for-You Plan? Try the Alignment Training Program

No more guessing what stretches to do or wondering if your workouts are reinforcing bad patterns.

Alignment Training is built around your specific Alignment Type

- Daily movements already laid out
- Breath and posture integrated into every session
- Designed to stabilize your core, correct imbalances, and support nervous system regulation
- Zero equipment required

Visit fxalign.com/reclaimvitality to receive 15 percent off your personalized ninety-day reset.

CHAPTER 19

Remove Toxic Inputs

We are not sick because of deficiencies in synthetic chemicals; we are sick because we are living outside our natural design.

—James Chestnut

The Virtue of Clean Living

We live in an industrialized world with multiplying exposure to toxins, but the goal isn't to fear the air we breathe or the food we eat. The goal is to understand the power of your body's ability to adapt and the value of living biologically congruent. That is the key to unlocking your body's ability to perpetually and effectively detox from the exposures of a twenty-first-century, industrialized life.

You can't avoid every toxin. But you can avoid creating your own toxic soup. And that begins with intentional rhythms that support the body's God-given design to adapt, heal, and cleanse. The great news is that each of the "R's" in this book support detoxification. This chapter is about how to *intentionally support detoxification* with rhythms and habits.

This chapter will help you identify hidden toxins in your daily life (pantry sweep, cosmetic sweep, home sweep) and implement the daily detox lifestyle that keeps your body adapting and removing daily exposures.

Detox Is Always Happening, but Is It Keeping Up?

Your liver, kidneys, lymphatic system, colon, lungs, and skin are constantly working to remove waste and toxins from your body. Of these, the liver is the primary organ responsible for converting fat-soluble toxins into water-soluble waste that can be excreted. It performs hundreds of essential functions and works in beautiful synergy with your gallbladder and lymphatic system. Lymphatic congestion is linked to systemic inflammation and impaired immunity. But this intricate detoxification network can become overwhelmed, especially when exposure outpaces elimination.

In our conversations with the Environmental Protection Agency (EPA), they have acknowledged that they have only recently started tracking endocrine disruption in a meaningful way. Their science is fifteen years behind simply because of the sheer amount of work and the regulatory processes that they have in place. That means we have to be our own gatekeepers. That's why reclaiming vitality means creating a lifestyle that reduces incoming toxins *and* supports daily, gentle detoxification. The best detox protocol isn't a three-day juice cleanse; it's how you live.

Toxic Effects Check-In (Circle all that apply in the past six months)

- Fatigue / low energy
- Brain fog
- Skin problems
- Sleep disruption
- Hormone imbalance
- Digestive issues
- Anxiety or mood swings

If you circled two or more, your toxic load may be impacting your body's ability to function at its best.

Step 1: Identify Toxic Inputs
Pantry Sweep: What's in Your Kitchen?
Instructions: Go to your pantry and fridge. Pull out the fifteen most used items from each. Check everything you find on the items' labels under ingredients. Now write down the items you're replacing immediately and the items you are replacing next time you go to the store.

1. Artificial Flavors and Colors
- Red 40 (Allura Red)
- Yellow 5 (Tartrazine)
- Yellow 6 (Sunset Yellow)
- Blue 1 (Brilliant Blue)
- Blue 2 (Indigo Carmine)
- Green 3 (Fast Green)
- "Artificial flavor" or "natural flavor" (often contains MSG or chemical solvents)

2. Artificial Sweeteners
- Aspartame (Equal)
- Sucralose (Splenda)
- Saccharin (Sweet'N Low)
- Acesulfame potassium (Ace-K)
- Neotame

3. MSG and Its Hidden Names *(Excitotoxins)*
- Monosodium glutamate (MSG)
- Hydrolyzed vegetable protein (HVP)
- Autolyzed yeast extract
- Calcium caseinate
- Soy protein isolate
- "Natural flavor" (often code for MSG)
- Disodium guanylate / inosinate

4. Harmful Oils and Fats
- Hydrogenated / partially hydrogenated oils (trans fats)
- Canola oil
- Soybean oil
- Corn oil
- Cottonseed oil
- Safflower oil
- Sunflower oil (unless high-oleic, cold-pressed)

5. Preservatives and Additives
- Sodium benzoate
- Potassium sorbate
- BHA (butylated hydroxyanisole)
- BHT (butylated hydroxytoluene)
- Propyl gallate
- TBHQ (tertiary butylhydroquinone)
- EDTA (calcium disodium EDTA)

6. Refined Sugars and Syrups
- High-fructose corn syrup (HFCS)
- Corn syrup solids
- Maltodextrin
- Dextrose
- Added sugars

7. Processed Meats *with* Nitrites/Nitrates
- Bacon (conventional)
- Hot dogs
- Lunch meats (ham, turkey, salami)
- Jerky

Action Step:
Write down **three items** you will throw away now:
1. _____
2. _____
3. _____

Action Step:
Write down **three items** you will swap next time you shop:
1. _____
2. _____
3. _____

<u>Cosmetic Sweep: What's in Your Bathroom or Makeup Bag?</u>
Instructions: Open your bathroom drawers, shower caddy, and makeup bag. Take out everything you currently use at least once per week. Check off any ingredient you see on your labels. Then, write down the products you'll replace this week.

1. Hormone Disruptors
- Parabens (methylparaben, propylparaben, butylparaben)
- Phthalates (often hidden under "fragrance" or "parfum")
- Benzophenone-3 (BP-3, oxybenzone—common in sunscreens)
- Octinoxate (ethylhexyl methoxycinnamate—sunscreen chemical)
- Triclosan (antibacterial soaps, toothpaste)

2. Heavy Metals
- Lead (lipstick, eyeliner—not listed on label, found in testing)
- Cadmium (lipstick, powders)
- Aluminum (antiperspirants, some cosmetics)
- Mercury (thimerosal in some eye makeup)

3. Harsh Surfactants and Foaming Agents
- Sodium lauryl sulfate (SLS)
- Sodium laureth sulfate (SLES)
- Ammonium lauryl sulfate

4. Preservatives and Formaldehyde-Releasers
- DMDM hydantoin
- Imidazolidinyl urea
- Quaternium-15
- Diazolidinyl urea
- Methenamine

5. Fragrances
- "Fragrance" or "parfum" (catch-all for hundreds of chemicals)
- Linalool

- Limonene
- Geraniol

6. Other Top Offenders
- Talc (especially untested for asbestos—in powders, blush, eyeshadow)
- Petrolatum / mineral oil
- Paraffin

Action Step: List the products you will replace this week with clean alternatives:

1. _____
2. _____
3. _____
4. _____
5. _____
6. _____

Household Cleaner and Laundry Sweep
Instructions: Go through your cleaning cabinet, laundry shelf, and anywhere you keep sprays, soaps, and detergents. Circle any ingredients you find. Write down the products you're ready to replace this week.

1. Common Toxins in Household Cleaners
- Bleach (sodium hypochlorite)—strong respiratory irritant, reacts with other chemicals to form toxic compounds
- Ammonia—can cause lung damage and eye irritation
- Quaternary ammonium compounds ("quats")—hormone disruptors, linked to asthma
- Phenols—toxic to liver and kidneys
- Formaldehyde—carcinogen used as a preservative in some cleaners
- Perchloroethylene (PERC)—dry-cleaning solvent, linked to cancer
- Fragrance/parfum—umbrella term for hundreds of untested chemicals, many of which are endocrine disruptors

- Chlorine—can cause skin and respiratory irritation; harmful in high exposure
- Volatile organic compounds (VOCs)—found in many sprays and polishes; contribute to indoor air pollution

2. Problem Ingredients in Laundry Products
- Fragrance/parfum—hidden chemicals that linger on clothing and bedding
- Optical brighteners—chemicals that make clothes look "whiter" by coating fabric with residue
- Phosphates—harmful to waterways and aquatic life
- Chlorine bleach—respiratory irritant; produces toxic by-products
- Nonylphenol ethoxylates (NPEs)—hormone disruptors banned in Europe, still used in some detergents
- Petroleum distillates—linked to nerve damage and respiratory issues
- Sodium lauryl sulfate (SLS)—skin irritant, can strip natural oils
- Benzyl acetate—linked to respiratory problems and possible carcinogenic effects

3. Problematic Disinfectants and Hand Sanitizers
- Triclosan—antibacterial agent linked to hormone disruption and antibiotic resistance
- Methanol—toxic alcohol found in some recalled hand sanitizers
- Synthetic fragrance—contains phthalates and allergens
- Chlorine-based sanitizers—can be harsh on skin and lungs
- Benzalkonium chloride (BAC)—skin and respiratory irritant

Safe Swaps
- ✓ Water and vinegar (4:1 ratio) for general cleaning
- ✓ Baking soda for scrubbing
- ✓ Castile soap (e.g., Dr. Bronner's)
- ✓ Essential oil sprays (tea tree, lemon, eucalyptus)
- ✓ Wool dryer balls with essential oils instead of dryer sheets
- ✓ Branch Basics, Norwex, Green Shield, and other clean brands

Action Step: List one cleaning product and one laundry product you will replace this week:

1. Cleaning product: _____

2. Laundry product: _____

EMF Home Audit Checklist
Principle: *Wired is for stationary use, wireless is for mobility.* —Odette Wilkens
Use this checklist to evaluate your home. Check off what you've already done and circle what you still want to tackle.

1. Go Wired Where You Can
   • Computers, TVs, and gaming consoles are plugged into Ethernet
   • Wi-Fi/Bluetooth disabled on devices that don't need them
   • Wi-Fi turned off whenever it's not in use, especially at night.
2. Use Phones Smarter
   • Use speakerphone or non-Bluetooth wired headset like airtubes (nonnegotiable!).
   • Phone not carried on the body (bras, waistbands, pockets), or shielded with a cell phone case.
   • Phone kept in another room, or in airplane mode while sleeping
   • Avoid long calls when signal strength is low (one to two bars)
3. Tame the Talkers
   • Replaced cordless (DECT) phone with corded model
   • Baby monitor is wired or used at a distance/off when not needed
   • Think twice before adding "Smart" appliances to the home; disable "smart" features (Wi-Fi/Bluetooth) on TVs/printers/appliances when possible
   • Router placed away from bedrooms/play areas

4. Miscellaneous High-Priority Cleanups
   - Whole-house dirty electricity filter
   - Use incandescent light bulbs
   - Opt out of a smart meter on your home; if unable to do so, do not spend a lot of time beside that place in your house and do not sleep next to it
   - Ditch your microwave, if you still have one

Bonus: Daily Grounding
   - Bare feet on grass/soil/sand at least fifteen minutes per day
   - Consider grounding mat for indoor use if outdoor time is limited

Step 2: The Daily Detox Lifestyle
Think of these five habits as biological requirements for supporting the brilliant design of the human frame. These five habits are some of your most affordable and fundamental tools of detox and should be a greater priority than expensive and complex detox protocols. Each habit keeps your detox pathways open and functioning so you can handle daily exposures.

1. Hydration: The Overlooked Cornerstone of Detox
Hydration isn't just about quenching thirst. It's the body's delivery system for detox. Water keeps drainage pathways and cells functioning, allowing toxins to leave through urine, sweat, breath, and stool. Every organ of detoxification, including the liver, kidneys, lymphatic system, and colon, depends on steady hydration. Without it, elimination slows, bile thickens, lymph stagnates, and immune function suffers.

You don't need a lab test to know if you're dehydrated: lingering pillow marks, dark urine, headaches, brain fog, or achiness are clear signs. The solution is simple yet powerful: drink clean, filtered water consistently throughout the day, not just when you're thirsty. Hydrating from within does far more for true antiaging than anything you could put on your skin.

Action Plan:

- Drink half your body weight in ounces daily
- Start your morning with a large glass of water and a pinch of sea salt or lemon to naturally support electrolyte balance and liver stimulation
- Remineralize any reverse-omosis-filtered water that you consume
- Avoid waiting until you're thirsty to drink your next glass of water
- Use a designated water bottle and track your intake

2. Antioxidant-Rich Foods

Free radicals damage cells. Antioxidants neutralize free radicals and protect your tissues.

A free radical is an unstable molecule that damages cells and accelerates aging. The average person's body takes over 10,000 oxidative hits per *cell* per day, and with over 50 trillion cells, the scale of damage is staggering. To counteract this, your body needs 12,000 mg of antioxidants daily, yet even a very healthy diet might provide only half that.

You can measure antioxidant intake in ORAC units (Oxygen Radical Absorption Capacity). The goal: 3,000–5,000 units per day. Most people get only 1,200–1,500. The solution? Eat the rainbow. Especially foods high in:

- **Anthocyanins** (blueberries, red cabbage)
- **Vitamin C** (kiwi, oranges, bell peppers)
- **Polyphenols** (green tea, dark chocolate, berries)

These nutrients help prevent your cells from moving through the five stages of decline: stressed, weakened, dysfunctional, mutated, diseased.

Certain foods and herbs actively support phase 1 and phase 2 liver detoxification:

- **Vegetables:** Asparagus, cabbage, celery, cucumbers, carrots, brussels sprouts, dark leafy greens
- **Fruits:** Watermelon, berries, pomegranate, citrus
- **Herbs:** Milk thistle, dandelion, turmeric, cordyceps
- **Special compounds:**
  - Green tea (catechins)
  - Broccoli and cauliflower (glucosinolates)

- Grapes (resveratrol)
- Watercress and pomegranate (ellagic acid)
- Hops (humulones)

These aren't "superfoods" for marketing purposes, they are therapeutic foods that actively aid the body's detox mechanisms.

3. Daily movement and Sweating

Your body was designed to move, and movement moves toxins. Your lymphatic system relies on muscle contractions to circulate and drain waste. Your skin eliminates toxins through sweat.

In generations past, sweating was a daily occurrence. Today, most people live at 70°F indoors and barely break a sweat.

Daily sweat goals: start a sweat calendar to check off each day that you sweated and write down the method used whether exercise, walking, running or sauna.

- Walk outside and get sunshine
- Use your big movers: quads, glutes, hamstrings
- Exercise until you sweat (twenty to forty minutes)
- Consider sauna therapy (preferably low-EMF or traditional)
- Hydrate before and after

Sweating supports the immune system, enhances detoxification, and reduces the body's toxic burden. Don't resent a fever, it's one of the body's most efficient ways to purge.

4. Proper Supplementation for Cellular Repair

These micronutrients help repair cellular damage and fuel detox pathways:

- Vitamins A, C, E
- Zinc, selenium, copper, manganese
- CoQ10
- Vitamin D_3 (supports immunity and cellular resilience)

Work with a trusted provider to ensure the right dosing and high-quality sourcing.

5. Faith over Fear

Chronic stress and fear keep your body in fight-or-flight, which shuts down detox. Choosing faith over fear, clarity over confusion, and ownership over outsourcing builds a life that is biologically aligned and emotionally empowered. Setting boundaries around toxic relationships, screen time, and cultural noise is as vital as filtering your water. Detox is about reclaiming inner and outer alignment because chronic stress impairs detox by keeping your body stuck in a survival state.

Nervous system interference comes from thoughts, traumas, and toxins. So we cannot talk about healing without talking about replacing our thoughts that keep us stuck in fear and stress. Gratitude changes your biology, and a peaceful heart supports a healing body.

Yes, we are exposed to more chemicals than any previous generation. But no, we are not helpless. God is not surprised by our modern world. He designed our bodies to be here for such a time as this and gave us the capacity to heal. Don't live like a victim of your environment. Take ownership. Steward your biology. Create an internal ecosystem of vitality.

Daily Practice:
- Gratitude journaling or speak aloud with your family before bed (list three daily).
- Prayer and meditation on what is true.
- Limiting toxic news and scrolling.

Assessing the Damage: Do You Need to Detox Beyond Daily Detox?

Tests can be helpful for some to understand the need for change. If you feel you need to test or want to test, a good practitioner can help you read and utilize testing. The Total Tox Burden test is a good place to start testing, if you have already removed known toxins and are still reacting to something in your environment. Total Tox Burden can show what exposures might still be lurking at home or at work by identifying heavy metals, mold toxins, and environmental chemicals. It is a self-administered urine test that highlights accumulation of toxins and exposures. You can find the Total Tox Burden test by visiting vitalitymetabolics.com/tests.

Start Assessing with a Long-Form Food Log

One of the best detox tests isn't a lab, it's a long-form food log. Even before you test, start with two weeks of a long-form food log and then remove the toxic exposures found on your food log from your diet for thirty days. So this is a six-week-long exercise.

Write down your top health concerns and how severe they are on a scale from one to ten on day one of your thirty-day reset (i.e., brain fog, achy joints, etc.) and then review those chief complaints and their severity after thirty days.

So you've probably seen food logs used by dietitians. This is a more detailed version: for two weeks, write down not just what you ate, but the *actual ingredients*. Don't just write down "chicken breast," but *where* the chicken came from and/or every ingredient listed on its label or on the restaurant's website. Was it from a regenerative farm or from a KFC combo meal? Was it prepared in canola oil or roasted in herbs? Unless you purchase the chicken from the farmer and cook it at home, who really knows if what you ate is just chicken and actually chicken.

If you eat out, look up the ingredients and write them down. Most chain restaurants have lists available online. You might discover hidden additives like monosodium glutamate (MSG), polysorbate 80, artificial colors, or hydrogenated oils that burden your liver.

This kind of audit will train your awareness and help you see patterns. It's also a powerful motivator: once you see what's going in, you'll be more motivated to clean it up.

Pro tip: If you feel guilty writing it down, it's probably something to rethink eating.

Pro tip 2: If you find yourself saying, "That wasn't typical," do another seven days and prove it.

Below are sample food logs that include common pitfalls. See if one of those looks like your typical day and then consider the suggested modifications.

The Sugar Burner Example (Estimated 2,800–3,200 kcal/day):
- **Breakfast:** Flavored yogurt (200 kcal), granola bar (250 kcal), orange juice (150kcal)
- **Snack:** Muffin (400 kcal), caramel latte (250 kcal)
- **Lunch:** Turkey sandwich on white bread (500 kcal), chips (200 kcal), soda (150 kcal)
- **Snack:** Candy bar (250 kcal)
- **Dinner:** Pasta with marinara sauce (600 kcal), garlic break (300 kcal), soda (150 kcal)
- **Late-Night Snack:** Ice cream (400 kcal)

Common Issue: High sugar intake and liquid calories cause insulin spikes and fat storage.

Suggested Modifications for the Sugar Burner (Approx. 1,800–2,000 kcal/day):
- **Breakfast:** Plain Greek yogurt with chia seeds and berries, black coffee or herbal tea (350 kcal)
- **Lunch:** Grilled chicken on organic greens with olive oil and balsamic vinegar, water with lemon (500 kcal)
- **Dinner:** Baked salmon with roasted broccoli and quinoa, water or herbal tea (600 kcal)
- **Snacking:** *Eliminated* to balance blood sugar and improve fat metabolism.

The Snacker Example (Approx. 2,600–3,000 kcal/day):
- **Breakfast:** Protein bar (150 kcal), banana (100 kcal), coffee with cream and sugar (120 kcal)
- **Snack:** Trail mix (300 kcal)
- **Lunch:** Chicken wrap (500 kcal), pretzels (200 kcal), iced tea (150 kcal)
- **Snack:** Smoothie (350 kcal), granola bar (200 kcal)
- **Dinner:** Stir-fry with rice (600 kcal), dark chocolate (200 kcal)
- **Snack:** Popcorn (250 kcal)

Common Issue: Frequent snacking keeps insulin elevated, blocking fat burning.

Suggested Modifications for the Snacker (Approx. 1,800–2,000 kcal/ day):

- **Breakfast:** Three scrambled eggs with avocado and spinach, black coffee (400 kcal)
- **Lunch:** Grilled chicken salad with olive oil dressing, water with lemon (500 kcal)
- **Dinner:** Grass-fed beef burger (lettuce wrap) with roasted veggies, herbal tea (600 kcal)
- **Snacking:** *Eliminated* to allow insulin levels to drop for fat burning.

The Carb-aholic Example (Approx. 2,800–3,200 kcal/day):

- **Breakfast:** Oatmeal with honey and raisins (400 kcal), toast with butter (200 kcal), orange juice (150 kcal)
- **Snack:** Granola bar (250 kcal)
- **Lunch:** Pasta salad (600 kcal), fruit juice (180 kcal)
- **Snack:** Crackers and cheese 300 kcal)
- **Dinner:** Pizza (2 slices, 600 kcal), salad with ranch (200 kcal), soda (150 kcal)
- **Late-Night Snack:** Cereal with milk (350 kcal)

Common Issue: Frequent snacking keeps insulin elevated, blocking fat burning.

Suggested Modifications for the Carb-aholic (Approx. 1,800–2,000 kcal/day):

- **Breakfast:** Scrambled eggs with avocado and sautéed greens, black coffee (400 kcal)
- **Lunch:** Grilled salmon with roasted vegetables, sparkling water (500 kcal)
- **Dinner:** Baked chicken thighs with Brussels sprouts and mashed cauliflower, herbal tea (600 kcal)
- **Snacking:** *Eliminated* to improve metabolic flexibility and fat adaptation.

Advanced Detox Steps: When you've implemented the rest and feel stuck
- ✓ Safely remove mercury fillings with a biological dentist
- ✓ Wear natural fiber clothing (cotton, wool)
- ✓ Drink detox teas (green tea, matcha, dandelion root)
- ✓ Test home for lead pipes or heavy metal plumbing
- ✓ Reduce EMF and radiation exposure
- ✓ Avoid living near coal-burning plants, fracking wells, or nuclear facilities

CHAPTER 20

Restore Alignment

The goal is simple: in your old age, you'll celebrate that you took care of your body, not regret that you neglected it.

—Dr. Mark Wolfman

The Virtue of Alignment

If you want to regulate the nervous system, you have to address spinal alignment.

Your nervous system doesn't just run on chemistry, it runs on communication. And that communication travels through your spine.

The Backbone of Alignment

Your spine is more than a stack of bones. It's the literal gatekeeper of your nervous system. Every organ, cell, and tissue in your body relies on signals traveling through the spinal cord. When the spine shifts out of alignment, those signals are distorted. It's simple but profound:

Structure affects function.
Alignment affects communication.

Misalignment can come from birth trauma, car accidents, poor posture, a bad mattress, or years of sitting. Each of these creates structural stress that alters proprioception, your body's sense of position. That stress ramps up inflammation and shifts your nervous system into a fight-or-flight state.

You might not feel pain right away, but your body feels the interference and stays on high alert.

That compensation comes at a cost. Digestion eventually slows down. Breathing becomes unconsciously shallower. Hormones go haywire. And muscles tighten in all the wrong places.

The solution isn't to "stretch it out" or "crack your own neck." You need to restore alignment and remove interference at the source. Because when structure is corrected, function is restored. And when the nervous system is balanced, the body heals.

Unlocking Neurological Potential

Neurospinal chiropractic isn't just about fixing posture or pain. It's about igniting the nervous system's capacity to heal, adapt, and transform.

1. Heart Rate Variability (HRV)

HRV measures how well your nervous system balances stress and recovery. A higher HRV indicates your body is better able to shift from stress mode into healing mode.

In a study covering over five hundred adults, just one chiropractic adjustment improved HRV. But after four weeks of care, those improvements held steady.[1] That means more calm, more control, and better stress management.

2. Brain Recharge

Heidi Haavik's research shows how adjustments alter brain activity in ways that matter. Scans show shifts in brain waves. Specifically, it shows less low-brain fog, more clarity, and better connection after adjustments. Over four weeks, chiropractic care also significantly improved subconscious sleep quality.[2]

In short: adjustments help brain patterns shift from fight mode to healing mode. That means sleep better, think clearer, or just feel overall more energy again.

3. Strength Shifts

Studies on stroke survivors found that a single chiropractic adjustment dramatically increased their muscle strength.[3] This happens thanks to changes in brain signals, not just muscle activation. That means adjustments don't just make your body move, they help your brain move your body better.

A Real-Life Patient Story

Keith didn't come to my clinic for back pain. He came in because his anxiety was horrible, and he hadn't slept more than five hours in months. Four weeks into neurologically based care, he said it out loud: "I feel like I got my brain back." He didn't expect chiropractic to fix his marriage or his mindset. But when your brain and body are in sync, things change.

Why This Matters for You

- **You're not stuck in stress mode.** Adjustments can shift your system into repair mode, so you recover faster, think sharper, and bounce back stronger.
- **You can physically feel the shift.** HRV improves. Sleep deepens. Strength returns.

The Most Underrated "Biohack" in the World

If neurospinal chiropractic care came in a bottle, it would be the bestselling "biohack" on the market. If it were a $400 wearable with sleek branding and influencer endorsement, everyone would have one. But it's not trendy. It's fundamental. It's been around for over a century without hype or hashtags.

Chiropractic care is the only health intervention that removes mechanical interference from the nervous system. Yet only a small fraction of the population is under consistent chiropractic care.

And that's a problem. If that were true for dental care, we'd see it everywhere with rampant decay, emergency extractions, gum disease. But we've normalized dental hygiene. We build it into the calendar. We teach our kids it's nonnegotiable.

The spine, the gateway to the nervous system, is treated like an afterthought. If you've read this far, you already know that's backward. Routine spinal care isn't a luxury. It's not just for people with back pain or neck tension. It's for anyone with a brain and a spine who wants to sleep better, recover faster, think clearer, move easier, and live with more energy.

Everyone deserves care that strengthens the most important system in the body. Not in an emergency. Not when things fall apart. But as a non-negotiable. As a way of life.

The Myth of Chiropractic Risk

My editor asked about the claim that chiropractic adjustments can cause a stroke, so I decided to address it here. This claim is one of the most persistent myths in healthcare. The truth is simple. Neck pain and headache are early signs of a vertebral artery dissection. People with those symptoms seek help. Some go to a chiropractor. Some go to a medical doctor. The stroke was already in motion before they arrived.[4]

The largest population study to date found no evidence of excess stroke risk from chiropractic care when compared to primary care. Both providers saw patients who were already developing a dissection.[5] Earlier studies that reported an association warned that the rarity of these events makes causation impossible to prove. Here is the bottom line. Chiropractic care, when done properly, is one of the safest interventions in all of healthcare.

You're Already Doing Nervous System Training

You're either reinforcing stress or restoring balance. Every time you sit hunched over your laptop, you're training your nervous system. Every time you ignore the tension, you're teaching your body to normalize it. But the same is true in reverse. Every adjustment, every breath, every aligned movement retrains your system to feel safe again.

The reality is that most of the structural breakdown doesn't happen from major traumas. It happens day-to-day. It's not the lifting of that object that wrecks your alignment. It's the way you sit, sleep, and slouch for hours that trains your body into dysfunction. The injury just highlighted the already existing dysfunction. Modern ergonomics are a slow-motion injury.

Let me give you some more examples:

- Stomach sleeping puts your neck in rotation for hours straight and compresses your low back. It's the fastest way to train misalignment while unconscious.
- Sitting for hours at a time shortens your hip flexors, deactivates your glutes, and stiffens your spine. Especially if you're sitting on a soft couch or sagging chair.
- Slouching at the desk pulls your shoulders forward, rounds your mid-back, and makes it nearly impossible to take a full breath.
- Tech posture, head down, arms forward, trains forward head posture and shifts the weight of your head from twelve pounds to over forty pounds of strain on your neck.

The nervous system responds to repetition. If your most consistent physical habits are collapsing your structure, don't be surprised when your body starts breaking down. But the same is true in reverse: every adjustment and every aligned movement retrains your system to feel safe again.

Write It Down:
Which of these daily patterns do you fall into?
- Do you sleep on your stomach?
- Do you sit for long stretches without moving?
- Do you regularly slouch at your desk, in the car, or on the couch?
- Do you spend hours looking down at your phone or laptop?
Circle the one that's most consistent in your life right now.

Ten-Second Nervous System Scan
You don't have to be in pain to be out of alignment. Pain is a lagging indicator. It shows up *after* interference has been building for weeks, months, or even years.

Misalignment often shows up in subtle, daily disruptions long before your body breaks down.

Check yourself:
Sleep and Energy
- Trouble falling or staying asleep
- Morning stiffness or grogginess
- Midday energy crash or brain fog

Mental State
- Racing thoughts when you try to relax
- Easily overwhelmed or emotionally reactive
- Feeling "on edge" even when life is calm

Physical Signs
- Tension headaches
- Shallow breathing
- Digestive issues (like bloating or irregularity)
- Cracking your own neck or back for relief

If you checked two or more, your nervous system is likely stuck in a low-grade stress response. These aren't random symptoms, they're early warning signs of neurological interference caused by spinal misalignment.

The good news? It's not permanent. Restoring alignment is more practical and more powerful than most people think.

Practical Rewire Actions: Unlock the System

1. Get Adjusted by a Neurologically Focused Chiropractor
This isn't about chasing cracks and pops. This is about restoring brain-body communication. A principled chiropractor trained in neurostructural correction doesn't adjust you just to feel good for five minutes, but to remove interference so your body can regulate for a lifetime.

Regular care = lower inflamma-tion, better stress response, better sleep, faster recovery, clearer thinking.

Find a neurologically based chiropractor at www.reclaimvitality.com/chiro.

2. Do Daily Spinal Hygiene (Wobble / Traction / Rolls)

Most people brush their teeth twice a day, but never care for their spine. Start wobbling on a balance disc. Use cervical traction to decompress your neck daily (especially after long screen sessions). Lay on rolls at night to help remold spinal curves. These are toothbrushes for your spine, preventative care that keeps the nervous system mobile and fluid.

Here are my videos teaching Spinal Hygiene. Check them out here:

> **Why Kids Need This Too (Start young, prevent breakdown)**
>
> *Kids fall. A lot. They stare at screens. They slouch in car seats. They're growing fast, and their nervous systems are wiring every day. And we didn't even talk about birth trauma. Adjustments aren't just safe for kids; they're one of the smartest things you can do to help your child develop without interference.*

Wobble [FxAlign.com/wobble] → Traction [fxalign.com/traction] → Rolls [fxalign.com/rolls]

3. Practice Alignment Training

You can't out-adjust poor posture. Alignment Training retrains how you move, sit, stand, and stabilize. It's not just about looking better, it's about moving better. Because when your movement is clean, your brain feels safe and healing happens.

Write It Down:
What postural pattern do you default to? Take the Alignment Type Quiz at fxalign.com/quiz

Awareness is the first step. Call it out.

Alignment Training Works Best with Chiropractic Care

Alignment Training is designed to support your nervous system by retraining posture, stabilizing movement, and reinforcing healthy spinal patterns. While it can be done on its own, the best and fastest results happen when it's integrated with neurologically based chiropractic care.

Adjustments remove interference. Alignment Training helps rewire how your body moves after that interference is cleared. One resets the signal. The other retrains the system.

---

4. Sleep in a Neutral Position

You already learned that sleep is repair time—but only if your body isn't twisted like a pretzel. Ditch stomach sleeping for good. Use a cervical roll under your neck and a firm pillow that supports spinal curves. Your spine needs restoration at night, not more tension.

Circle This:

Stomach sleeper? Side sleeper? Back sleeper?

Now circle which one actually supports your spinal alignment (hint: it's *not* stomach).

5. Move in Alignment

It's time to retire the crunch. Most traditional ab workouts reinforce the same patterns that cause misalignment. Instead, build your core through bracing, glute activation, and spinal stability. Again, a lot of this is accomplished through Alignment Training, but those same movements must transfer to daily life: bending, lifting, squatting, walking, breathing.

Write It Down:

What's one movement you repeat often (picking up the kids, working, training)?

How can you make that movement more aligned?

Barriers to Watch For

- **Ignoring chronic tension or "nagging" postural pain:** Your body whispers before it screams. Listen closely.
- **DIY "Adjustments" or Cracking Your Own Neck:** You might feel a release, but you're reinforcing instability. Stop calling it an "adjustment." It's not. And it's a sign you need a real one.
- **Sleeping with Too Many Pillows or No Neck Support:** It's seven to eight hours of positional retraining. Be intentional. Use the spinal molding rolls found at www.fxalign.com to help.

Write It Down:
Which of these barriers do you currently face?
Circle the one that needs to change first.
What small action can you take *today* to start correcting it?

CHAPTER 21

Metabolism, Weight Loss, and the Energy Equation

The Virtue of Food Temperance

Contributor Spotlight: Dr. Ryan Sousley

For this chapter, I've invited my good friend and colleague, Dr. Ryan Sousley, to join me. I didn't bring him in just because of his deep expertise in metabolic health, although he is one of the most knowledgeable doctors and educators I know. I brought him in because I have had the privilege of watching him live these principles for more than a decade.

Ryan is not just a clinician; he is a walking case study in what a hot-burning metabolism looks like in real life. He and his family embody consistency, strength, and health at the highest level. When it comes to energy, fitness, and metabolic mastery, he is not just teaching it, he is living it.

Together, we want to help you see metabolism for what it truly is and give you the tools to keep yours running at full capacity for life.

Dr. Ryan Sousley

My journey into health optimization started in my adolescence as an athlete. I played several competitive sports like football, basketball, and baseball, and the higher up in sports I got, the more I started looking for a competitive edge. I found it in nutrition and other holistic lifestyle practices including chiropractic, mobility work, sleep optimization, and mindset training. After graduating high school as an all-state first team quarterback, I went on to play college football, and my pursuit of health optimization and human performance grew exponentially. I proceeded to earn a bachelor's degree in exercise science and then a doctorate in chiropractic in order to practically share my knowledge and expertise with others.

Since then, I have completed several full- and half-distance Ironman triathlons and ultra-endurance races in order to test my mettle and the science of human performance that I continue to pursue to this day. But beyond athletic performance, I've learned during my journey that human performance and health optimization is not just about being able to compete as an athlete, but more importantly to be able to show up as your fullest self for those you love and care about most.

We all have a God-given purpose in life, and whether you're competing as an athlete, raising a family, or contributing to society through your work, your performance and production are directly proportional to your level of health. For me, the driving force behind health optimization and human performance has transcended athletics, and is now about being able to show up as the man I want to be for my wife and four kids, for my patients who look to me as the standard, and my community, which is counting on my contribution and leadership in our ever increasingly challenging world. So my goal for this chapter is to educate and empower you with science and strategy to elevate and improve your metabolism, but not just lose weight, improve function, and feel better in your body (although I can almost guarantee you will if you take action), but to enable you to fully pursue your purpose and build a life that benefits others and a legacy that you can be proud of.

Metabolism Is a Health Issue

When we talk about metabolism, most people immediately think of burning calories or shedding a few pounds. But your metabolism isn't just about the number on the scale. It's about how your body produces energy, heals, fights disease, and keeps you sharp and vibrant every single day.

Think about it. Have you ever felt exhausted for no reason? Struggled with brain fog? Had poor sleep? Dealt with stubborn digestive issues or hormonal swings?

That's metabolism, too. Your metabolism controls how fast or slow you age, how well you recover from stress, how strong your immune system is, and how clearly your brain functions. It's the engine behind your energy, focus, and resilience. It's like a sluggish car battery. Even if there's nothing wrong with the components or equipment, your car will never function optimally, and will eventually break down, because the individual parts and systems aren't getting the power they need to thrive.

So even if you don't need to lose a pound, the real questions are: How do you feel? How are you functioning? And how long can you keep feeling and functioning this way? Because a strong metabolism doesn't just keep you lean, it keeps you young. It keeps you vital. And it keeps you living fully.

Metabolism is directly tied to blood pressure, cholesterol, heart disease, type 2 diabetes, cancer, autoimmune conditions, thyroid conditions, and more. Unfortunately, 88 percent of Americans have a metabolic disorder and most don't even know it.[1] The

> **Circle This**
>
> Rate yourself from 1 to 10 in these areas (1 = poor, 10 = optimal):
>
> - Energy throughout the day
> - Mental claity
> - Sleep quality
> - Recovery after stress or exercise
> - Waist circumference/ weight stability
>
> Now circle the ONE area you most want to improve over the next 30 days.

signs are everywhere and often normalized. The afternoon crash, the belly fat that won't budge, waking up tired, living on caffeine or sugar just to function, and that constant, low-grade puffiness and inflammation you've almost convinced yourself is "just aging" are all signs of metabolic distress.

Write It Down

Which of these have you noticed in yourself? Afternoon crashes, stubborn belly fat, waking up tired, constant cravings, puffiness, or swelling.

List them here: _____

Now put a star next to the one that affects your life the most.

Metabolic distress is initiated by more than just overeating. Some of the biggest offenders are:

- **Chronic stress**—keeps your body in fight-or-flight, raising cortisol and storing more fat.
- **Ultra-processed "Food by Man"**—spikes blood sugar, inflames the gut, and derails hormones.
- **Sedentary lifestyle**—signals your body to burn fewer calories and preserve fat.
- **Poor sleep**—wrecks insulin sensitivity and appetite regulation.
- **Toxic load**—environmental chemicals and pesticides that stress the liver and slow fat metabolism.

Fat Cells Become Toxic

Excess toxins get stored in fat cells, and those fat cells behave like an organ. Fat tissue produces estrogen through a process called aromatization, which converts testosterone into estrogen. The more body fat you carry, the more your hormones tip in the wrong direction, leading to fatigue, muscle loss, stubborn weight, and in some cases, increased cancer risk.

This is why testosterone replacement therapy (TRT) and other quick-fix hormone treatments are a joke when it comes to restoring hormone health. If you're still carrying the excess body fat that's feeding the hormonal imbalance, all you're doing is throwing expensive gas on a fire you haven't put out. Hormone therapy without fixing metabolism is a temporary mask for a deeper dysfunction. And it will likely create a liability in your journey to reclaim vitality.

Here's the wild part about fat cells: once they get overfed and inflamed, they don't just sit quietly expanding your waistline, they go full gossip mode. Hypertrophic (bloated) fat cells start releasing chemical messengers, like exosomes loaded with a protein called caveolin1, which literally reprogram neighboring stem cells to become *more fat cells*.[2] It's like a toxic mentorship program. On top of that, the longer you stay in that inflamed metabolic state, the more your fat tissue undergoes epigenetic changes, basically flipping genetic switches that favor storing fat, slowing your metabolism, and making weight loss harder.[3] And even if you lose the weight? Some of those changes stick around, setting the stage for rebound weight gain.[4] So yes, toxic fat can *teach your body to stay fat.* But the good news? With the right strategy, you can unlearn that biology and rewire it for fat loss and performance.

Circle This

Of these metabolism disruptors (chronic stress, ultra-processed food, sitting too much, poor sleep, toxin exposure), which one is your biggest obstacle?

Now write the ONE change you will make this week to address it:

The Elephant in the Room: Weight-Loss Drugs

Before we dive into the natural tools that actually heal your metabolism, let's talk about the current craze: GLP-1 Weight-Loss drugs like Ozempic, Wegovy, and Mounjaro. These have taken the world by storm, marketed as the miracle fix for stubborn fat. And yes, the number on the scale moves, but it is a game of metabolic roulette. Endocrine and organ function is manipulated and hijacked, creating a cascade of problems that obesity may or may not have caused.

GLP-1 is a hormone your body naturally produces after eating. It helps regulate blood sugar, suppress appetite, and promote fat metabolism. These drugs mimic that hormone, but here's the kicker: they don't fix anything. They override your biology, rather than repair it. Think of it like turning off your smoke alarm without putting out the fire.

Research shows up to 40 percent of the weight lost on GLP-1 drugs is lean muscle,[5] not fat, and muscle is the metabolic engine you *don't* want to lose. Less muscle means a slower metabolism, lower energy, and a higher likelihood of regaining the weight once the meds stop. Add to that the side effects (nausea, bloating, digestive issues, thyroid concerns), and the trade-off becomes clear: you're shrinking your body but not actually getting healthier.

As Dr. Jason Fung explains in *The Obesity Code*, weight gain is driven by hormonal imbalances, insulin resistance, and cellular dysfunction, not just willpower or calories.[6] And GLP-1 drugs? They don't address the root causes. They simply mute the symptoms.

But here's the good news, your body *already knows how* to activate GLP-1 naturally. You just need to give it the right inputs:

- **Protein- and fiber-rich foods** (like wild salmon, pastured eggs, lentils, and leafy greens) naturally stimulate GLP-1 and keep you full longer.
- **Strength training and HIIT** boost GLP-1 production while also building the muscle that keeps your metabolism firing.
- **Targeted supplements** can support GLP-1 activity without the side effects—and unlike drugs, they come with bonus benefits like improved digestion, hormone balance, and cellular energy.

So instead of outsourcing your biology to a prescription, what if you reclaimed it? In the next section, we'll break down the best natural GLP-1 activators to help you lose fat, build energy, and reset your metabolism for the long haul, without sacrificing your muscle, your health, or your bank account.

Write It Down
Describe in one or two sentences what a "hot-burning metabolism" would look and feel like in your life.

Example: "I wake up energized, think clearly, and recover quickly. My body stays strong and lean year-round without extreme diets."

Yourstatement:_____

Red-Hot Metabolism

Muscle is your metabolic engine. It burns calories around the clock, even when you're sleeping. In fact, research shows that each pound of muscle burns six to ten calories per day at rest, while fat tissue burns only about two.[7] So the more muscle you have, the more fat you burn doing absolutely nothing.

Let's put that into perspective: if you gained just two pounds of lean muscle, your body would burn an extra 120–200 calories per day, without changing anything else. That adds up to twelve to twenty pounds of fat burned over a year, just by building a little more muscle and letting your metabolism do the work.

But it doesn't stop there. Muscle also improves insulin sensitivity, meaning your body can process carbohydrates more efficiently instead of shuttling them into fat storage. It enhances mitochondrial function, the energy-producing machinery in your cells, which helps every system in your body, from your brain to your hormones, run better.[8]

The problem? Most people lose muscle as they age, not because of age itself, but because they stop challenging their bodies. Reverse that trend, and you *reverse the clock*. Strength training isn't just about looking fit. It's a direct investment in your metabolism, hormone balance, bone density, and longevity. When you pair it with strategic fasting, you turn your body into a fat-burning, energy-producing, age-defying machine.

Muscle isn't just for performance. It's your insurance policy for a longer, leaner, stronger life.

Write This Down

I commit to _____ days per week of strength training for the next thirty days.

Write down the exact days/times you'll do it:

_____

Fasting for Metabolism Optimization

Done strategically, fasting is one of the most powerful tools to reset your metabolism. It lowers inflammation, improves insulin sensitivity, and triggers a process called autophagy, the cellular cleanup and repair that keeps your systems running efficiently.

Intermittent fasting isn't a trend, it's a return to how the human body was designed to function. For most of human history, food wasn't available 24/7. Our ancestors naturally cycled between periods of eating and fasting based on hunting, gathering, and seasonal availability. This rhythm trained the body to burn fat for fuel, repair damaged cells, and regulate hormones efficiently. In fact, modern research shows that fasting activates powerful metabolic pathways, like autophagy and insulin sensitivity, that are hardwired into our physiology. Fasting is a way of syncing with your original blueprint.

Fasting also supports mitochondrial health by giving your body a break from constant digestion so it can focus on repair and regeneration. You don't have to jump into extreme fasting windows. Even a daily twelve-to-sixteen-hour fast between dinner and your first meal the next day can make a profound difference.

Time-restricted eating isn't about starving yourself until noon. It's about creating a long enough overnight break from food so your body can lower insulin, repair cells, and shift into fat-burning mode. That "fast" starts when you finish your last meal of the day. If you finish dinner at 6:30 p.m. and eat your first meal at 8:30 a.m., you've already fasted fourteen hours, without skipping breakfast.

The key is that when you do break your fast, you break it right. Start your eating window with a nutrient-dense, protein-rich "Food by God" so you're fueling recovery, not just cutting calories. The high protein aspect signals your body to preserve muscle, stabilize blood sugar, and switch smoothly from fasting mode to fuel-burning mode. You can have the best of both worlds by:

- Ending dinner earlier to extend your fast overnight.
- Breaking your fast with 25–40g of protein (or 0.6–0.8g per pound of ideal body weight divided over the day).

This keeps all the benefits of fasting while making sure you aren't sacrificing muscle or tanking your metabolism. In order to achieve this, you'll need to have specific eating windows. These are your "time-restricted eating" windows.

Write It Down
Choose your starting eating window:
- Twelve hours
- Ten hours
- Eight hours
- Six hours

I'll commit to trying it _____ days this week.

**Note from Nick: I started with an eight-hour eating window on most days of the week several years ago. I now incorporate one twenty-four-hour fast per week (Dinner on Sunday to Dinner on Monday) in conjunction with weekly time-restricted eating windows. This has been the best rhythm for long-term sustainability for me.

Clean Carb Cycling for Metabolic Flexibility

Your body is designed to be metabolically flexible, able to switch efficiently between burning carbs for quick energy and fat for long-term fuel. Think about it like a car that is able to burn both gasoline and diesel depending on its situational demands, and you would get the best of both worlds. Your metabolism is designed to operate in this manner, but most people lose this flexibility due to constant high-carb intake, insulin resistance, and a sedentary lifestyle. That's where Clean Carb Cycling comes in. It's a strategic way to restore metabolic adaptability, improve energy levels, and support body composition without wrecking your hormones.

On rest or low-activity days, lowering your carb intake encourages your body to shift into fat-burning mode and increase insulin sensitivity. On training or high-output days, adding in clean, nutrient-dense carbs helps refuel glycogen stores, enhance workout recovery, and support thyroid and hormone function.

A 2018 study in *Cell Metabolism* found that switching between low- and high-carb states helps maintain mitochondrial efficiency and improves metabolic resilience.[9] Another study from the *Journal of Nutrition and Metabolism* showed that carb cycling may reduce fat mass and increase lean body mass compared to a consistent calorie-restricted diet.[10]

The key is not eating the same way every day but matching your carb intake to your energy demand. Clean carbs, what we call "Food by God," include things like sweet potatoes, berries, squash, bananas, quinoa, and wild rice. These whole-food sources come packed with fiber, antioxidants, and minerals that support healthy blood sugar and gut health, unlike the processed carbs that tank your energy and trigger cravings.

Bottom line: Carb cycling is about precision fueling. It's a smart choice.

When done right, it helps you train harder, recover faster, burn more fat, and regain control of your metabolism.

The De-Stress Your Metabolism Action Plan

- **Morning sun and movement**—Ten to fifteen minutes of natural light and light movement within thirty minutes of waking.
- **Front-load protein**—0.6–0.8g per pound of ideal body weight per day, divided over meals. At least one-third of your daily target at first meal.
- **Strength first**—Full-body training 3x/week, never more than two days off.
- **Time-restricted eating**—Six-to-twelve-hour eating window (5+ days/week).
- **Carb cycling**—Lower carbs on rest days, clean carbs on training days.
- **Sleep like your life depends on it**—Seven to nine hours/night.
- **Hydrate and mineralize**—Half body weight in ounces of water and electrolytes.

When you follow the de-stress plan, you're more than "boosting metabolism," you're fortifying your energy, resilience, and vitality for decades to come. The goal is to incorporate all seven and make it habitual.

Write it down:
1. Which disruptor from earlier is your biggest challenge?
2. Which ONE action from the Daily Metabolism Protocol will you commit to for the next seven days?
3. How will you measure your win at the end of the week?

CHAPTER 22

The Truth about Lab Testing and Supplements

Supplements aren't magical. But in a devitalized world, they are necessary.

—Unknown source

The Virtue of Nonintervention

There's a difference between *intervening* and *supporting*. The more we try to override the body, the more we tend to interfere with it. That's the principle behind the Virtue of Nonintervention—**to limit outside-in treatments and allow healing from within.**

This isn't about doing nothing. It's about doing the right *less*.

Intervention exists on a spectrum. On one end, you have ten medications managing twelve symptoms that all stem from the same root cause. On the other end, you have someone living simply, eating well, and thriving with no need for outside help. Both extremes are real, but few of us live at the edges.

The tension is this: You want to heal from within. But the world you live in makes pure nonintervention more difficult. That's why I don't give everyone twenty pills a day. And I don't tell them to tough it out with nothing, either.

My job is to help you navigate that tension. To restore what's been stolen. To remove the interferences. To give your body enough support to reclaim its design.

This is how you begin to exit the conventional model. Not by trading prescriptions for supplements. But by restoring what your body needs so it can stop outsourcing its health to a system that never taught you how to heal.

So when someone asks me, *"What should I be taking?"* I don't give them a shopping list. I help them build a strategy.

You can't supplement your way out of a toxic lifestyle. But you also can't ignore what your body is missing.

Food is always first. Consistency matters. But if you're living in the twenty-first century, you're already swimming upstream. The soil is depleted. Environmental and emotional stressors are relentless. Toxins are unavoidable. And your body, especially your nervous system, is trying to operate on fumes.

What You're Up Against

It's not just that you're tired, inflamed, or foggy. It's that your cells are missing what they need to function.

Compared to even one hundred years ago, your baseline nutrient load is down. Magnesium has been stripped from the soil. Omega-3s are outcompeted by inflammatory seed oils. Vitamin D production is blocked by sunscreen, long winters, and desk jobs. And that's before we even talk about B-vitamins, amino acids, or trace minerals.

This is the modern paradox:

We're overfed and undernourished. We've got more food but less nutrition. More stress but fewer reserves. You can eat clean, sleep well, move daily and still be depleted. That's modern life.

Why Foundational Support Comes First

Before chasing symptoms with trendy protocols, you need to fill the gaps. We start with what we call Foundational Support, the five key nutrients your body needs every single day to function, heal, and adapt. These are the five most important but also the most commonly depleted nutrients in our modern world.

We package this into something called Daily Essentials:

- **Vitamin D$_3$ and K$_2$**—for immune strength, inflammation control, and calcium regulation
- **BioAvailable magnesium**—to calm your nervous system, stabilize blood sugar, and support muscle and brain function
- **Essential omega-3s**—to balance inflammation, protect your brain, and support hormones
- **B-complex**—for energy, methylation, detox, and stress response
- **Gender-specific multivitamin**—to cover micronutrient gaps based on your unique physiology

This is your foundation. It's like running your home on full power instead of flickering lightbulbs. These resources can be found on vitalitymetabolics.com.

No matter what your goal is, better sleep, more energy, hormone support, or nervous system repair, these nutrients make it possible. Without them, reclaiming vitality becomes an uphill battle.

Circle This: Which of these five are you currently taking daily?
Vitamin D$_3$ and K$_2$
BioAvailable magnesium
Essential omega-3s
B-complex
Gender-specific multivitamin

Quality > Hype
Not all supplements are created equal. The industry is flooded with garbage. Cheap fillers, low absorption forms, and formulas that are more marketing than true fulfillment.

Here's what we look for in quality:

- **Bioavailability**—Is your body actually able to absorb it? A supplement is different from food. It needs to work.

- **Purity**—Free from dyes, binders, and synthetic garbage. In our toxic world, this is critical.
- **Backed by research**—Not just influencer trends. Unfortunately, many of the influencer-marketed supplements are lacking in this department.

Every product we use is professional grade. That means clinical dosing, third-party testing, and formulations that match human physiology, not hype cycles.

Strategic Supplementation

Start with the foundation of Daily Essentials. Then, layer in targeted support based on your story:

- **Fatigue or brain fog?** Could be a magnesium or CoQ10 deficiency. CoQ10 deficiency is very common, especially if you've taken a statin medication.
- **Chronic stress?** Adaptogens like ashwagandha, rhodiola, or l-theanine can be very helpful in allowing your body to adapt.
- **Poor sleep?** Could be a magnesium or glycine deficiency. Could also be a dysregulation of neurotransmitters. The Reset PM formula is designed to help with all of the above.
- **Toxic burden?** If you believe you are toxic, adding in cleansing nutrients can be very helpful. I like the product called InflammaBalance, as it is a blend of botanicals, antioxidants, and amino acids that support phase 1 and phase 2 liver detox. You can find it at vitalitymetabolics.com.

Supplements work best when they match your physiology, not just your Instagram feed. Outside of the foundational support, supplements are not lifelong crutches. They're temporary scaffolding to rebuild your health. You can't outsource your healing. But you can support it.

Supplement Strategy Guide: What to Take and When

Step 1: Build Your Base
If you're not taking these daily, start here and then *layer in based on how you feel.*
- **BioAvailable magnesium**
- **Vitamin D$_3$ and K$_2$**
- **Essential omega-3s**
- **B-complex**
- **Gender-specific multi**

These five form the foundation of energy, sleep, focus, hormone balance, and inflammation control.

Step 2: Target the Interference
Circle the area that fits your current challenge:
If you're tired all the time . . .
Start with:
- **B-complex** (if already taking, increase dose)
- **CoQ10** (especially if you've taken statins)
- **Adrenal adaptogens** (like ashwagandha or Rhodiola)

Also consider:
- Magnesium at night (helps with restorative sleep)

If your stress or anxiety feels chronic . . .
Start with:
- **Magnesium** (twice daily, typically)
- **L-theanine** or **GABA support**
- **Adaptogens** (holy basil, ashwagandha, rhodiola)

Also consider:
- Reset PM if stress is affecting sleep

If you're not sleeping well . . .
Start with:
- **Magnesium** One to two hours before bed
- **Glycine** (calms brain, promotes deep sleep)

- **Reset PM** (blend of calming herbs, nutrients, and neurotransmitter support)

Also consider:

- Blue light blockers and earlier dinners (not a supplement, but critical)

If your digestion is off (bloating, constipation, reflux) . . .

Start with:

- **Digestive enzymes** (with every meal)
- **Serum IgG support** (to calm inflammation)
- **Spore-based probiotic** (after two to four weeks of gut repair)

Also consider:

- GI repair nutrients (glutamine, aloe, zinc carnosine)

If you have joint pain, inflammation, or brain fog . . .

Start with:

- **Omega-3s** (minimum 2g daily EPA/DHA)
- **InflammaBalance**
- **Turmeric or curcumin complex**

Also consider:

- Magnesium and Vitamin D to calm systemic inflammation

If you suspect mold, toxin overload, or chemical sensitivity...

Start with:

- **ToxiBind** (binder that grabs and escorts toxins out)
- **InflammaBalance** (liver support and antioxidants)
- **Glutathione support** (optional—start slow)

Also consider:

- Detox-friendly foods: cruciferous vegetables, lemon water, grass-fed protein

Step 3: Still unsure? Then test.

If multiple areas overlap, or symptoms aren't budging, it's time for targeted testing. Start with one:

- Nutrient panel

- Gut test
- Hormone or adrenal panel
- Toxin test (mold, metals, chemicals)

Write this down:
What's your **next right step?**
(Choose one to start. Don't try to do it all.)

Gut Repair: Don't Just Take Probiotics

Gut healing isn't a one-size-fits-all probiotic. It's a layered strategy. If your gut is inflamed, leaky, or under constant attack, no amount of healthy food or supplements will get absorbed properly. That's why we often start with GI supportive nutrients before anything else.

Here's the order:

- **Digestive enzymes**: Help break down food properly and take the stress off your gut.
- **Serum IgG support**: Binds to pathogens and toxins, reducing gut inflammation. Also helps with repairing the gut lining.
- **GI repair nutrients**: Think of this as topical nutrition for your gut lining—glutamine, aloe, and botanicals that help seal the leaks.
- **Spore probiotics**: Survive stomach acid and train your immune system, unlike most store-bought strains. They also won't feed into short-intestinal bacterial overgrowth (SIBO). If you've ever taken probiotics and felt worse, you might have SIBO. This is why we save probiotics for last. Heal the terrain first, then reinoculate.

Stop Wasting Money On . . .

You don't need a supplement graveyard. Here's what to skip, or at least rethink:

1. Multivitamins from the grocery store

Most are made with cheap forms of nutrients your body can't absorb.

They're produced by the same companies that make soda and candy bars. Not a joke.

2. Isolated "miracle" nutrients
Taking turmeric by itself while you're inflamed, depleted, and constipated? That's like throwing a match on wet wood and expecting a bonfire.

3. Collagen without gut support
Collagen doesn't repair a leaky gut if you're still inflamed and eating junk. It's a Band-Aid until the foundation is in place.

4. Gummies and powders packed with fillers
Artificial sweeteners, food dyes, and processed additives wreck your microbiome. You're paying for flavor, not function.

5. Detox teas and "cleanse kits" from influencers
If there's no binder, no drainage support, and no lifestyle changes, it's not a detox. It's a diuretic.

6. Generic probiotics
Most die before they ever reach your gut. If you want real impact, use spore-based strains and pair with gut repair.

7. Supplements with synthetic folic acid or cyanocobalamin
Especially if you have MTHFR or methylation issues, these forms backfire. Choose methylated B_{12} (methylcobalamin) and folate (5-MTHF).

Bottom line: If it's cheap, mass-produced, and marketed like candy, it's probably garbage.

Strategic Testing: Test, Don't Guess
Here's the reality: You don't need a lab test to know if you're exhausted, inflamed, or not sleeping.

But when you've hit a wall or when symptoms aren't responding, testing becomes highly useful. Specialty lab tests help us identify:
- **Nutrient deficiencies**

- **Gut infections or leaky gut**
- **Hormone imbalances**
- **Toxic load (mold, metals, chemicals)**
- **Metabolic dysfunction**

The right test at the right time gives clarity and saves time. It lets you stop guessing and start solving. But testing is only valuable when it's used in service of vitality restoration, not just adding supplements to manage symptoms. Unfortunately, many specialty lab tests are now being used for tracking or data collecting purposes.

Write This Down: What do you actually want to know?
Testing without intention leads to overwhelm. But clarity comes when you name the question.

What's one question you'd like testing to help answer?

(Examples: "Is my fatigue nutrient-related?" "Do I have gut damage?" "Is mold impacting my nervous system?")

Circle This: What kind of test might help you answer it?
- Nutrient Panel
- Gut / Stool Test
- Hormone Panel
- Toxin (Mold, Metals, Chemical)
- Inflammation / Autoimmune
- Unsure—need help deciding

Behind the Lab Coat: The Truth about Corporate Labs and Data

There's a growing obsession with tracking everything. Your steps, your sleep, your HRV, your blood sugar, your microbiome, all of it are being gamified. At first glance, this seems empowering. But this data feeds algorithms built with intentions of influence and control.

You might think of Quest Diagnostics and LabCorp as neutral testing companies. But these aren't mom-and-pop operations, they're two of the largest data brokers in the healthcare system, with deep ties to pharmaceutical companies, insurance giants, and government agencies.

Here's what most people don't realize:

1. Your Labs Are Not Just for You

Once your lab work is processed, the results don't just go into your chart. They go into massive data lakes, aggregated, analyzed, and sold. These companies openly market their de-identified data to biotech, insurance, and government partners.

LabCorp owns Covance, one of the largest drug development companies in the world. Quest has long-standing contracts with federal agencies, including the CDC and Department of Defense. Make no mistake, these tests are widely accessible, because it's not just about your health. It's about using your biology to drive profit, policy, and population-level algorithms.

2. Function Health and the Rise of Full-Spectrum Surveillance

We are concerned about other companies that position themselves as "the future of preventive medicine." Mark Hyman's Function Health is one example. Function Health is backed by Andreessen Horowitz (a16z), a venture capital firm whose vision for the future goes far beyond better lab testing.[1]

Marc Andreessen, the firm's founder, is a vocal supporter of AI-driven governance, transhumanism, and what he calls "e-governance," the idea that digital systems, not traditional governments, should shape the rules of society. Andreessen Horowitz actively invests in infrastructure projects tied to biometric surveillance, digital identity, and World Economic Forum–aligned biotech initiatives.

In this model, your health data isn't just data. It's your passport, your scorecard, and your potential chain. Function Health might look like personalized wellness. But its financial backbone is deeply aligned with a vision that sees the human body as a digitally managed asset, not a sovereign creation.

What they don't tell you is that you're also building a permanent biometric file, blood chemistry, heart rate, sleep patterns, and soon, genetic data.

Who owns that file? Not you. Read the fine print and you'll see that your data can be used for research and development, shared with third-party partners, and stored indefinitely in cloud-based systems that are vulnerable to breach or misuse.

This is the medical wing of the Surveillance Economy. This is what Catherine Austin Fitts calls "digital slavery." A system where your biology becomes a barcode, your health status is trackable, and access to care, employment, or insurance can be manipulated based on your score.

3. Health Is the Trojan Horse

Fitts has warned for years that control systems are being built under the guise of care. Digital IDs, vaccine passports, and biometric monitoring are all being normalized in the name of safety or prevention. Lab testing is the perfect front. It feels scientific, empowering, and personal. But if you're not careful, you're voluntarily uploading your body into a database you can't control and can never escape.

Test Strategically

We're not anti-testing. We're antislavery. Testing should serve your health, not harvest your data. That's why we:

- Use labs strategically, not as a default or subscription
- Refuse wearables or platforms that stream data to cloud servers
- Avoid labs that bundle data into third-party databases
- Partner only with labs that respect patient sovereignty and transparency

You are not a data point. You are not an input for someone else's AI. Your health decisions should remain between you, your family, and God who designed your body, not algorithms run by biotech-funded mega-corporations.

To find out which specialty labs we currently support, you can go to dr-wilson .com/tests for an up-to-date list.

CHAPTER 23

Redefining the Win

Count it all joy, my brothers, when you meet trials of various kinds, for you know that the testing of your faith produces steadfastness. And let steadfastness have its full effect, that you may be perfect and complete, lacking in nothing.

—James 1:2–4 (ESV)

I was told when writing this book to only include the things I was certain about. The truths I know deep in my heart and believe will stand the test of time. That became the filter for every chapter.

Before we close, I need to leave you with something that may be the most important truth of all. It will not just change how you respond to sickness or stress. It will reshape how you process your daily experiences:

Even when it does not work out the way you hoped, it's still for you.
I've watched good people do everything right. They ate clean, got adjusted, moved their bodies, and aligned their lives with purpose. They stewarded their health with discipline, not out of fear but out of faith. And still, they got the diagnosis.

Sometimes it happens fast. Stage 4, aggressive, gone in months. Those moments can shake everything. You start to question whether any of it mattered. Did the choices make a difference, or were we clinging to a false sense of control?

It's not easy to sit with those questions. I've mourned with friends and families who lost loved ones far too soon. I've stood bedside as their worst fears unfolded. But somewhere in that pain, a deeper truth surfaced. The goal was never to eliminate all suffering. The win was never a perfect body or a "clean bill of health." The win was how they lived. Fully alive, faithful, and unshaken. They knew that along the journey, each hiccup, each hurdle, each detour was *for* them. For their good. For their protection. Nothing was wasted.

They weren't scrambling at the end to make peace or course correct. They had already chosen peace long before the battle began. They had built something internal that disease couldn't take. That's what health really is.

Health is not the absence of discomfort or diagnosis. If that's your definition, fear will rule your life. You'll chase perfection, panic at symptoms, and feel like a failure when things go sideways. That kind of mindset produces bondage and captivity, as we talked about in the early chapters of this book.

True health is about how you respond, how you adapt, and how deeply you're rooted when the storm comes. It's not about dodging every illness or pain. It's about living in a way that honors your design, stewarding your body well, and listening to the signals that guide you back to wholeness. That's what vitality really means.

You won't find that kind of resilience in formulas or quick fixes. It's built through conviction and lived experience. It's true nervous system regulation, not nervous system protection. It's spiritual grounding, not symptom avoidance. Real health is revealed when pressure comes. Do you collapse in fear or rise in faith? That's the better measure.

Reframe the Win

What was your old definition of health? Was it about being pain-free, diagnosis-free, always "on track"? Cross it out and write a new one. Health is the ability to recover quickly, live with peace, have light in your eyes, walk uprightly, and stay grounded in truth no matter what I face.

Circle that sentence. Let it reframe how you measure progress from this point forward. Because setbacks will come. But your posture in the face of them, that's the real test.

This way of life doesn't promise ease. It doesn't guarantee the outcome you hoped for. It guarantees that you won't be owned by fear when the outcome surprises you. And yes, the by-product of honoring God's design and living in alignment with natural order is that you gain a true reference point. A compass. You'll begin to see through the noise. You'll fall for fewer tricks, fewer tests, and fewer empty promises. Over time, I'm convinced you'll become more of a noninterventionist because of pure awe. Awe at how the body can adapt, heal, and recover, even in our imperfection. That's faith and wisdom that can only be developed through experience.

I've seen people walk through death with more dignity and peace than some people bring into life. That's not because they escaped struggle. It's because they were rooted before the storm ever came. That's what we're after.

Once you step into this new way of thinking, you stop doubting the signals. You stop fearing your body. You see that what's happening is happening *for* you. Every symptom, even the hard things, can become a teacher, not a threat. Genetic changes that seemed like a curse may have been what protected you and allowed life to continue. You don't know the full story yet, but you can trust the One who does. When you accept this, you don't panic at symptoms, and you don't outsource every decision to someone in a white coat. You begin to live with peace. Even when it's hard, even when it doesn't make sense at the moment, your default becomes trust. Trust in the design. Trust in the process. Trust that even this is for your benefit. That's health freedom.

You may still get sick. You may face something hard. But it won't define you or rob you of your faith. You'll have something deeper than, and foundational to, physical health. You'll have peace. You'll have purpose. And that is the win.

You've made it this far, and that matters more than you know. Not just because you finished a book, but because you chose to question the system, lean into a new way of thinking, and take ownership of your life: how you live, how you show up, how you heal, and how we pass on principles of health and freedom to our children. That takes courage. That takes conviction.

This isn't the end. It's a new beginning. A turning point in your journey to reclaim what was always yours: vitality, freedom, and the unshakable peace that comes from living in alignment with how you were created.

My hope is that this book was more than information, but that it was a spark. A reminder of the strength already placed inside you and the courage that comes with faith in the design.

Thank you for trusting us with your time, your attention, and your health. I don't take it lightly. I hope when we see each other in the community that we recognize the light in each other's eyes and we are mutually reminded to keep going, keep growing, and enjoy the journey on the path to reclaim vitality.

In health and freedom,
Dr. Nick and Leah Wilson

Who do you know who needs this book? Gift them a copy by visiting the website of your local or a preferred national bookseller.

Notes

Chapter 2

1   Martin A. Makary and Michael Daniel. 2016. "Medical Error—the Third Leading Cause of Death in the US," *BMJ* 353: i2139.

2   Ibid.

3   Barbara Starfield. 2000. "Is US Health Really the Best in the World?" *Journal of the American Medical Association* 284, no. 4: 483–485.

4   Gary Null, Carolyn Dean, Martin Feldman, Debora Rasio, and Dorothy Smith. 2010. "Death by Medicine," *International Journal of Health Services* 40, no. 1: 1–14.

5   Peter C. Gøtzsche. 2013. *Deadly Medicines and Organised Crime: How Big Pharma Has Corrupted Healthcare* (London: Radcliffe Publishing).

6   Joanna Moncrieff. 2008. *The Myth of the Chemical Cure: A Critique of Psychiatric Drug Treatment* (New York: Palgrave Macmillan).

7   U.S. Department of Health and Human Services. July 2021. *Confronting Health Mis-information: The U.S. Surgeon General's Advisory on Building a Healthy Information Environment.*

8   Mark Zuckerberg, interview by *New York Post.* January 10, 2025. "Biden Officials Screamed at Meta Execs to Take Down Vaccine Posts."

9   Lucian L. Leape. 1994. "Error in Medicine," *Journal of the American Medical Association* 272, no. 23: 1851–1857.

10 John T. James. 2013. "A New, Evidence-Based Estimate of Patient Harms Associated with Hospital Care," *Journal of Patient Safety* 9, no. 3: 122–128.

11 E. Richard Brown. 1979. *Rockefeller Medicine Men: Medicine and Capitalism in America* (Berkeley: University of California Press).

12 Ibid.

13 Ibid.

14 Abraham Flexner. 1910. *Medical Education in the United States and Canada: A Report to the Carnegie Foundation for the Advancement of Teaching* (New York: Carnegie Foundation).

15 Ibid.

16 Brown, *Rockefeller Medicine Men.*

17 Ibid.

18 Ibid.

19 Ibid.
20 Centers for Disease Control and Prevention, *Antibiotic Resistance Threats in the United States, 2019* (Atlanta: CDC, 2019).
21 World Health Organization, *Global Antimicrobial Resistance and Use Surveillance System Report, 2021* (Geneva: WHO, 2021).
22 Münevver Demir Joerdens, Tom Luedde, and Karel Kostev 2022. "Antibiotic Therapy Is Associated with an Increased Incidence of Cancer," *Journal of Cancer Research and Clinical Oncology.*
23 Thomas McKeown. 1976. *The Role of Medicine: Dream, Mirage, or Nemesis?* (Princeton: Princeton University Press).
24 U.S. Census Bureau. 1975. *Historical Vital Statistics of the United States.*
25 John Colgrove. 2002. "The McKeown Thesis: A Historical Controversy and Its Enduring Influence." *American Journal of Public Health* 92 (5): 725–729.
26 Ibid.
27 CDC. "Chronic Diseases in America." Centers for Disease Control and Prevention. Accessed November 12, 2025. https://www.cdc.gov/chronic-disease /data-research/facts-stats/index.html.
28 National Cancer Institute, SEER Cancer Statistics Review, 1975–2019.
29 Ibid.
30 Richard Nixon, "State of the Union Address," January 22, 1971.
31 Gøtzsche, *Deadly Medicines.*
32 Tom Nichols. 2017. *The Death of Expertise: The Campaign Against Established Knowledge and Why It Matters* (New York: Oxford University Press).
33 *The Holy Bible*, Galatians 5:19–21 (NRSV), James Strong, *Strong's Exhaustive Concordance of the Bible*, entry for *pharmakeia.*
34 *The Holy Bible*, Revelation 18:23 (NRSV).
35 U.S. Department of Justice, "The Opioid Epidemic: By the Numbers," DOJ, 2019.
36 Moncrieff, *The Myth of the Chemical Cure.*
37 HHS, *Confronting Health Misinformation.*
38 Uffe Ravnskov. 2000. *The Cholesterol Myths: Exposing the Fallacy That Saturated Fat and Cholesterol Cause Heart Disease* (Washington, DC: New Trends Publishing).
39 CDC, *Antibiotic Resistance Threats in the United States, 2019.*
40 HHS, *Confronting Health Misinformation.*
41 Pew Research Center, "COVID-19 and Alternative Medicine Attitudes," Pew, 2021.
42 U.S. Food and Drug Administration, "FDA Approves Sovaldi for Hepatitis C," Press Release, December 6, 2013.
43 Gilead Sciences, *Annual Report 2017.*
44 Goldman Sachs, *The Genome Revolution: Is Curing Patients a Sustainable Business Model?* (Goldman Sachs Investment Research, April 10, 2018).
45 CMS, *Medicare Benefit Policy Manual, Chapter 16—General Exclusions from Coverage.*

46 Ibid.

Chapter 3

1   Louis Pasteur. 1878. "Germ Theory and Its Applications to Medicine and Surgery" in *The Foundations of Microbiology* (New York: Appleton, 1923).

2   Claude Bernard, quoted in Hans Selye, *The Stress of Life* (New York: McGraw-Hill, 1956), 15.

3   G. T. Evans, E. A. Repasky, and D. T. Fisher. 2015. "Fever and the Thermal Regulation of Immunity: The Immune System Feels the Heat," *Nature Reviews Immunology* 15, no. 6: 335–349.

4   Simon Szreter. 1988. "The Importance of Social Intervention in Britain's Mortality Decline, 1850–1914," *Social History of Medicine* 1, no. 1: 1–38.

5   J. W. Hurst. 1946. "Occupational Asthma Due to Pyrethrum," *Journal of the American Medical Association* 130, no. 4: 240–243.

6   W. C. Jordan. 1911. "Experimental Production of Colds," *Journal of Infectious Diseases* 9, no. 2: 190–200.

7   J. Douwes, P. Thorne, N. Pearce, D. Heederik, and I. R. Douglas. 2003. "Bioaerosol Health Effects and Exposure Assessment: Progress and Prospects," *Annals of Occupational Hygiene* 47, no. 3: 187–200.

8   Patrick Forterre. 2010. "Defining Life: The Virus Viewpoint," *Origins of Life and Evolution of the Biosphere* 40, no. 2: 151–160.

9   Eugene V. Koonin and Tatiana G. Senkevich. 2013. "Origins and Evolution of Viruses of Eukaryotes: The Ultimate Modular Organisms," *Annual Review of Microbiology* 67: 341–362.

10 Frank Ryan. 2009. *Virolution* (New York: HarperCollins).

11 J. R. Dowling and W. G. Winter. 1963. "Lack of Transmission of the Common Cold Under Controlled Conditions," *American Journal of Epidemiology* 77, no. 1: 91–101.

12 Milton Rosenau. 1919. "Experiments to Determine Mode of Spread of Influenza," *Journal of the American Medical Association* 73, no. 5: 311–313.

13 Tom Jefferson et al. 2023. "Physical Interventions to Interrupt or Reduce the Spread of Respiratory Viruses," *Cochrane Database of Systematic Reviews* 1: CD006207.

14 Ibid.

15 "Physician Defies Contagion Belief," *Wisconsin State Journal*, March 12, 1903.

16 Milton Rosenau. 1919. "Experiments to Determine Mode of Spread of Influenza," *JAMA* 73, no. 5: 311–313.

17 J. C. Ray. 1970. "Outbreak of Influenza in an Isolated Antarctic Base," *British Medical Journal* 4, no. 5688: 587–589.

18 Peter Doshi. 2010. "Pandemic Influenza: Lessons from Remote Communities," *BMJ* 340: c292.

19 Francisco J. Ayala. 2016. "Viruses as Evolutionary Agents," *Proceedings of the National Academy of Sciences* 113, no. 24: 6731–6738.

20 Kenneth W. Witwer and Clotilde Théry. 2014. "Extracellular Vesicles and

Exosomes: Definition, Isolation, and Research Priorities," *Current Protocols in Cell Biology* 103, no. 1: 3–22.

21 Luis P. Villarreal. 1997. "Viruses and the Evolution of Life," *American Scientist* 85, no. 5: 440–450.

22 Maya J. Wei et al. 2014. "Herpes Zoster and Risk of Glioma," *BMC Medicine* 12: 28.

23 Ziyad Al-Aly et al. 2023. "Tumor Regression Following Severe COVID-19: Case Series," *Frontiers in Oncology* 13: 117.

24 Stephen J. Russell et al. 2014. "Remission of Disseminated Cancer after Systemic Oncolytic Virotherapy," *Mayo Clinic Proceedings* 89, no. 7: 926–933.

25 Joseph Wiemels et al. 2009. "History of Chickenpox and Risk of Glioma: A Report from the UCSF Adult Glioma Study," *Cancer Research* 69, no. 17: 6870–6874.

26 Suzanne Garland. 2019. "Childhood Infections and Reduced Cancer Risk," *International Journal of Cancer* 144, no. 5: 1013–1024.

27 Suzanne Simard. 2012. "Mycorrhizal Networks: Mechanisms, Ecology and Modelling," *Fungal Biology Reviews* 26, no. 1: 39–60.

28 Martha K. McClintock. 1971. "Menstrual Synchrony and Suppression," *Nature* 229, no. 5282: 244–245.

29 Zach Bush. n.d. "Virome Replay," accessed August 27, 2025, https://zachbushmd.com/virome-replay/.

30 Charles C. Horn. 2006. "Why Is the Neurobiology of Nausea and Vomiting So Important?" *Appetite* 46, no. 3: 355–358.

31 "Illness Expectations Predict the Development of Influenza-like Symptoms," *Journal of Psychosomatic* Research 133 (October 2020): 110128.

32 "Worry Kills More than the Disease," *Chicago Tribune*, October 12, 1918.

33 Sheldon Cohen et al. 2006. "Positive Emotional Style Predicts Resistance to Illness After Experimental Exposure to Rhinovirus or Influenza A," *Psychosomatic Medicine* 68, no. 6: 809–815.

34 Naomi Oreskes and Erik M. Conway. 2010. *Merchants of Doubt* (New York: Bloomsbury), on fear as a driver in medicine and public health.

Chapter 4

1 World Medical Association, "WMA Declaration of Helsinki—Ethical Principles for Medical Research Involving Human Subjects," last amended 2013.

2 Centers for Disease Control and Prevention, Advisory Committee on Immunization Practices (ACIP), October 2024 Meeting Summary, https://www.cdc.gov/vaccines/acip/meetings/index.html.

3 Nayu Ikeda et al. 2011. "What Has Made the Population of Japan Healthy?" *Lancet* 378, no. 9796: 1094–1105.

4 World Health Organization. 2023. "World Health Statistics 2023: Monitoring Health for the SDGs." Geneva: WHO.

5 Centers for Disease Control and Prevention, "Immunization Schedules: Birth–18

Years," 2023, https://www.cdc.gov/vaccines/hcp/imz-schedules/child-adolescent -age.html.

6   Marian F. MacDorman et al. 2016. "Trends in Infant Mortality in the United States, 2005–2014," NCHS *Data Brief* no. 279. Hyattsville, MD: National Center for Health Statistics.

7   Amy J. Houtrow et al. 2014. "Changing Trends of Childhood Disability, 2001–2011," *Pediatrics* 134, no. 3: 530–538.

8   Institute of Medicine. 2013. *The Childhood Immunization Schedule and Safety: Stakeholder Concerns, Scientific Evidence, and Future Studies*. (Washington, DC: National Academies Press).

9   National Center for Health Statistics. 2968. *Vital Statistics Rates in the United States, 1940–1960* (Washington, DC: Government Printing Office).

10   Thomas McKeown. 1979. *The Role of Medicine: Dream, Mirage, or Nemesis?* Princeton: (Princeton University Press).

11   U.S. Congress, House of Representatives, Hearings before the Subcommittee on Health of the Committee on Interstate and Foreign Commerce, Testimony of Dr. Bernard Greenberg, July 1962.

12   Nita Vashisht and Jacob Puliyel. 2012. "Polio Programme: Let Us Declare Victory and Move On," *Indian Journal of Medical Ethics* 9, no. 2: 114–117.

13   Ritu Dhiman. 2018. "Correlation between Non-Polio Acute Flaccid Paralysis Rates with Pulse Polio Frequency in India," *International Journal of Environmental Research and Public Health* 15, no. 5: 898; S. Awasthi et al. 2016. "Increase in Non-Polio Acute Flaccid Paralysis Cases in India," *Indian Pediatrics* 53, no. 1: 57–60.

14   Jane S. Smith. 1990. *Patenting the Sun: Polio and the Salk Vaccine* (New York: William Morrow).

15   U.S. Congress, House of Representatives, Hearings before the Subcommittee on Health of the Committee on Interstate and Foreign Commerce, Testimony of Dr. Bernard Greenberg, July 1962.

16   U.S. Department of Health and Human Services, "CARES Act Provider Relief Fund: General Information," 2020; Centers for Medicare & Medicaid Services, "COVID-19 Emergency Declaration Blanket Waivers for Health Care Providers," 2020. The Council of State and Territorial Epidemiologists' April 15, 2020 position paper for defining what constitutes a COVID case—without implementing safeguards to ensure that single individuals would not be counted multiple times, thus altering case counts and subsequent data; Minnesota State Senator Dr. Scott Jensen told Laura Ingraham on April 8: "Right now Medicare has determined that if you have a COVID-19 admission to the hospital, you'll get paid $13,000. If that COVID-19 patient goes on a ventilator, you get $39,000, three times as much."

17   Centers for Disease Control and Prevention, "Vaccine Excipient Summary," 2023, https://www.cdc.gov/vaccines/pubs/pinkbook/downloads/appendices/B /excipient-table-2.pdf.

18 See, for example, U.S. Food and Drug Administration, Package Insert, "MMR-II (Measles, Mumps, and Rubella Virus Vaccine, Live)," 2018, sec. 13.1.

19 U.S. Food and Drug Administration, "Package Insert, Engerix-B (Hepatitis B Vaccine)," 2019, sec. 13.1.

20 Institute of Medicine. *The Childhood Immunization Schedule and Safety* (2013).

21 *Bruesewitz v. Wyeth LLC*, 562 U.S. 223 (2011).

22 Code of Federal Regulations, Title 21, sec. 201.57 (2020).

23 U.S. Food and Drug Administration, "Package Insert, Gardasil 9 (Human Papillomavirus 9-valent Vaccine)," 2020, sec. 6.

24 Ross Lazarus et al. "Electronic Support for Public Health—Vaccine Adverse Event Reporting System (ESP:VAERS)." Final Report. Harvard Pilgrim Health Care, 2011.

25 Vaccine Adverse Event Reporting System (VAERS), "VAERS Data," 2018, https://vaers.hhs.gov/data.html.

26 National Childhood Vaccine Injury Act of 1986, Pub. L. 99–660, 100 Stat. 3755.

27 Health Resources and Services Administration, "National Vaccine Injury Compensation Program Data Report," 2023.

28 Centers for Disease Control and Prevention, "Historical Immunization Schedule, 1995–1999," https://www.cdc.gov/vaccines/schedules/hcp/imz/child-adolescent.html.

29 Centers for Disease Control and Prevention, "Immunization Schedules: Birth–18 Years," 2023.

30 Coleen A. Boyle et al. 2011. "Trends in the Prevalence of Developmental Disabilities in U.S. Children, 1997–2008," *Pediatrics* 127, no. 6: 1034–1042.

31 Centers for Disease Control and Prevention, "Most Recent National Asthma Data," 2023.

32 Kathleen R. Merikangas et al. 2010. "Prevalence and Treatment of Mental Disorders among U.S. Children in the 2001–2004 NHANES," *Pediatrics* 125, no. 1: 75–81.

33 Matthew J. Maenner et al. 2023. "Prevalence and Characteristics of Autism Spectrum Disorder among Children Aged 8 Years—Autism and Developmental Disabilities Monitoring Network, 11 Sites, United States, 2020," *MMWR Surveillance Summaries* 72, no. 2: 1–14.

34 World Health Organization, "Measles and Rubella Strategic Framework 2021–2030," Geneva: WHO, 2020.

35 Texas Department of State Health Services, "Measles Investigation Update, 2024."

36 Pierre Kory, interview with author, March 2024.

37 National Center for Health Statistics, *Vital Statistics Rates in the United States, 1940–1960*.

38 Lawrence Palevsky, interview in *The Truth about Vaccines* (docuseries, 2017).

39 Irja Davidkin et al. 2006. "Persistence of Measles, Mumps, and Rubella

Antibodies in an MMR-Vaccinated Cohort: A 20-Year Follow-Up," *Journal of Infectious Diseases* 194, no. 6: 756–762.

40 Hiroshi Kawashima et al. 2000. "Detection and Sequencing of Measles Virus from Peripheral Mononuclear Cells from Patients with Inflammatory Bowel Disease and Autism," *Digestive Diseases and Sciences* 45, no. 4: 723–729.

41 Matthew J. Maenner et al. 2023. "Prevalence and Characteristics of Autism Spectrum Disorder among Children Aged 8 Years—Autism and Developmental Disabilities Monitoring Network, 11 Sites, United States, 2020," *MMWR Surveillance Summaries* 72, no. 2: 1–14.

42 H. Albonico et al. 2008. "Infectious Diseases and Cancer: The Paradox of the Measles," *Medical Hypotheses* 70, no. 5: 1012–1016.

43 Christopher A. Shaw and Lucija Tomljenovic. 2013. "Aluminum in the Central Nervous System: Toxicity in Humans and Animals, Vaccine Adjuvants, and Autoimmunity," *Immunologic Research* 56, no. 2–3: 304–316.

44 U.S. Health Resources and Services Administration, "National Vaccine Injury Compensation Program Data Report," 2023.

45 See deposition of Dr. Andrew Zimmerman, *Hazlehurst v. Secretary of HHS*, No. 03–654V (Fed. Cl. 2018).

46 Paul Fine et al. 2011. "Herd Immunity: A Rough Guide," *Clinical Infectious Diseases* 52, no. 7: 911–916.

47 Centers for Disease Control and Prevention, "Global Polio Eradication Initiative: Vaccine-Derived Polioviruses," 2022.

48 Global Advisory Committee on Vaccine Safety, "OPV and Shedding Risks," *WHO Weekly Epidemiological Record* 95, no. 25 (2020): 301–312.

49 Centers for Disease Control and Prevention, "Vaccine Withdrawals and Discontinuations," 2022.

50 Lucija Tomljenovic and Christopher A. Shaw. 2013. "Human Papillomavirus (HPV) Vaccine Policy and Evidence-Based Medicine: Are They at Odds?" *Annals of Medicine* 45, no. 2: 182–193.

51 Centers for Disease Control and Prevention, ACIP Meeting Minutes, September 2021.

Chapter 5

1 Caleb E. Finch. 2007. *The Biology of Human Longevity: Inflammation, Nutrition, and Aging in the Evolution of Lifespans* (San Diego: Academic Press), 214–220.

2 Francis S. Collins et al. 2003. "A Vision for the Future of Genomics Research," *Nature* 422, no. 6934: 835–847.

3 Teri A. Manolio et al. 2009. "Finding the Missing Heritability of Complex Diseases," *Nature* 461, no. 7265: 747–753.

4 Shing Wan Choi and Paul F. O'Reilly. 2019. "Polygenic Risk Scores: From Research Tools to Clinical Instruments," *Nature Reviews Genetics* 20, no. 9: 581–590.

5 National Institute of Environmental Health Sciences (NIEHS), "Genes and the Environment," accessed August 27, 2025. https://www.niehs.nih.gov/health/topics/science/genetics.

6   Tuuli Lappalainen and Ewan Birney. 2014. "Genetic Architecture: Polygenic Inheritance and the Complex Interactions of Genes and Environment," *Nature Reviews Genetics* 15, no. 9: 591–600.

7   Nancy L. Pedersen et al. 2002. "The Swedish Twin Registry in the Third Millennium: An Update," *Twin Research and Human Genetics* 5, no. 5: 427–432.

8   Kaare Christensen et al. 2002. "The Danish Twin Registry: A Unique Resource for Epidemiological Research," *Journal of Internal Medicine* 252, no. 4: 310–314.

9   James W. Vaupel et al. 2003. "Genetics of Human Longevity," *Science* 299, no. 5611: 1320–1321.

10 University of Oxford. "Lifestyle and Environmental Factors Affect Health and Ageing More Than Our Genes." News, February 20, 2025. https://www.ox.ac .uk/news/2025–02-20-lifestyle-and-environmental-factors-affect-health-and -ageing-more-our-genes.

11 Dorret I. Boomsma et al. 2002. "The Netherlands Twin Register: Longitudinal Research Based on Twin and Family Studies," *Twin Research and Human Genetics* 5, no. 5: 401–406.

12 Gonneke Willemsen et al. 2010. "The Netherlands Twin Register Biobank: A Resource for Genetic Epidemiological Studies," *Twin Research and Human Genetics* 13, no. 3: 231–245.

13 Nancy L. Pedersen et al. 1989. "Does Cardiovascular Disease Run in Families? Twin and Adoption Studies of Heart Disease and Related Disorders," *Acta Geneticae Medicae et Gemellologiae* 38, no. 3–4: 333–345; Nancy L. Pedersen et al. 1991. "Genetic and Environmental Factors in the Etiology of Cardiovascular Disease: A Twin Study," *Atherosclerosis* 91, no. 1–2: 1–10; Nancy L. Pedersen et al. 1998. "Genetic Influences on Cardiovascular Risk Factors: Results from the Swedish Adoption/Twin Study of Aging," *Journal of Gerontology: Medical Sciences* 53A, no. 1: M59–M65; A. Rissanen et al. 1991. "BMI and Obesity in Twins Reared Apart: Results from the Swedish Adoption/Twin Study of Aging," *International Journal of Obesity* 15, no. 9: 673–681.

14 Elmar W. Tobi et al. 2009. " DNA Methylation Differences after Exposure to Prenatal Famine Are Common and Timing- and Sex-Specific," *Human Molecular Genetics* 18, no. 21: 4046–4053.

15 Rebecca C. Painter et al. 2008. "Transgenerational Effects of Prenatal Exposure to the Dutch Famine on Neonatal Adiposity and Health in Later Life," *BJOG: An International Journal of Obstetrics & Gynaecology* 115, no. 10: 1243–1249.

16 Peter S. Harper. 1996. *Huntington's Disease*, 3rd ed. (London: W.B. Saunders).

17 Ahmad Al-Mrabeh et al. 2019. "Hepatic Lipoprotein Export and Remission of Human Type 2 Diabetes," *Cell Metabolism* 30, no. 2: 267–276.e4.

18 Robert A. Waterland and Randy L. Jirtle. 2003. "Transposable Elements: Targets for Early Nutritional Effects on Epigenetic Gene Regulation," *Molecular and Cellular Biology* 23, no. 15: 5293–5300.

19 LC Hartmann et al. 1999. "Efficacy of Bilateral Prophylactic Mastectomy in Women with a Family History of Breast Cancer," *NEJM* 340: 77–84.

20 Nature Research, "The Angelina Jolie Effect," *NPJ Breast Cancer* 7, no. 10 (2021). https://pmc.ncbi.nlm.nih.gov/articles/PMC7854742/.

21 MD Anderson Cancer Center. "BRCA and Your Cancer Risk: What You Need to Know," *Focused on Health*, MD Anderson Cancer Center, accessed October 4, 2025.

22 J. M. Hall, M. K. Lee, B. Newman, J. E. Morrow, L. A. Anderson, B. Huey, and M.-C. King. 1990. "Linkage of Early-Onset Familial Breast Cancer to Chromosome 17q21," *Science* 250, no. 4988: 1684–1689.

23 Anthony C. Antoniou et al. 2003. "Average Risks of Breast and Ovarian Cancer Associated with BRCA1 or BRCA2 Mutations Detected in Case Series Unselected for Family History: A Combined Analysis of 22 Studies," *New England Journal of Medicine* 349, no. 19: 1299–1308.

24 Aimé Nkondjock and Pierre Ghadirian. 2008. "Nutritional Risk Factors for Breast Cancer: A Case-Control Study among French-Canadian Women," *International Journal of Cancer* 123, no. 3: 653–660.

25 Sunita Desai et al. 2015. "Rise in BRCA Testing after Angelina Jolie's Disclosure: An Interrupted Time Series Analysis," *JAMA* 314, no. 6: 617–624.

26 Karoline B. Kuchenbaecker et al. 2013. "Modifiers of Cancer Risk in BRCA1 and BRCA2 Mutation Carriers: Systematic Review and Meta-analysis," *JAMA* 310, no. 4: 385–396.

27 Dean Ornish et al. 2005. "Intensive Lifestyle Changes May Affect the Progression of Prostate Cancer," *Journal of Urology* 174, no. 3: 1065–1070.

28 Hilary A. Tindle, et al. 2007. "Optimism, Cynical Hostility, and Incident Coronary Heart Disease and Mortality in the Women's Health Initiative," *The Lancet* 370, no. 9596: 1605–1611.

29 Bradley P. Turnwald, et al. 2019. "Learning One's Genetic Risk Changes Physiology Independent of Actual Genetic Risk," *Nature Human Behaviour* 3, no. 1: 48–56.

30 Sheldon Cohen, et al. 2012. "Chronic Stress, Glucocorticoid Receptor Resistance, Inflammation, and Disease Risk," *Proceedings of the National Academy of Sciences* 109, no. 16: 5995–5999.

31 Stephen F. Kingsmore et al. 2019. "A Genome Sequencing System for Universal Newborn Screening, Diagnosis, and Precision Medicine," *Genetics in Medicine* 21, no. 1: 68–77.

32 U.S. Food and Drug Administration, *Orphan Drug Act: Frequently Asked Questions*, updated 2022.

33 M. L. Escolar et al. 2005. "Krabbe Disease: One Hundred Years from the Bedside to the Bench to the Bedside," *Journal of Neuroscience Research* 79, no. 5–6: 583–590.

34 Sheryl Gay Stolberg. November 28, 1999. "The Biotech Death of Jesse Gelsinger," *New York Times*.

35 Asher Mullard. 2019. "FDA Approves Gene Therapy for Spinal Muscular Atrophy," *Nature Biotechnology* 37, no. 6: 575–576. "Retraction Note: Rescue of

the Spinal Muscular Atrophy Phenotype in a Mouse Model by Early Postnatal Delivery of SMN," *Nature Biotechnology* 40, no. 11 (November 2022): 1692.

36 Jacob S. Sherkow. 2021. "Illumina, BGI, and the Race for genomics IP," *Nature Biotechnology* 39, no. 5: 499–501.

37 Joel E. Bialosky et al. 2005. "The Influence of Spinal Manipulation on Oxidative Stress and DNA Repair: Serum Thiol Levels in Long-term Chiropractic Patients," *Journal of Vertebral Subluxation Research* 1, no. 1: 1–7.

Chapter 6

1 Richard Nixon, "Special Message to the Congress Proposing a National Health Strategy," *Public Papers of the Presidents of the United States*, December 9, 1971.

2 National Cancer Institute, *SEER Cancer Statistics Review, 1975–2019*, Surveillance, Epidemiology, and End Results Program, 2021.

3 National Cancer Institute, *Surveillance, Epidemiology, and End Results (SEER) Program*. "Lifetime Risk of Developing or Dying of Cancer." Updated 2024. Accessed October 4, 2025. https://seer.cancer.gov/statistics/types/lifetimerisk.html.

4 National Research Council, *DDT, Human Health, and the Environment* (Washington, DC: National Academies Press, 1975).

5 Linda S. Birnbaum. 2012. "Environmental Chemicals: Evaluating Low-Dose Effects," *Environmental Health Perspectives* 120, no. 4: a143–a144.

6 Michele Carbone et al. 1998. "Simian Virus 40, Poliovirus Vaccines and Human Tumors: A Review of Recent Developments," *Oncogene* 17: 3065–3077.

7 Ivan Illich. 1975. *Medical Nemesis: The Expropriation of Health* (New York: Pantheon Books).

8 Barry M. Popkin. 2001. "Nutrition in Transition: The Changing Global Nutrition Challenge," *Asia Pacific Journal of Clinical Nutrition* 10, no. S1: S13–S18.

9 Abraham Flexner. 1910. *Medical Education in the United States and Canada: A Report to the Carnegie Foundation for the Advancement of Teaching* (New York: Carnegie Foundation).

10 Michael Retsky et al. 2013. "Postsurgical Promotion of Metastasis: A Critical Review," *Cancer Research* 73, no. 8: 2413–2423.

11 Isaiah J. Fidler. 2003. "The Pathogenesis of Cancer Metastasis: The 'Seed and Soil' Hypothesis Revisited," *Nature Reviews Cancer* 3, no. 6: 453–458.

12 Romano Demicheli et al. 2008. "The Effects of Surgery on Tumor Growth: A Century of Investigations," *Annals of Oncology* 19, no. 11: 1821–1828.

13 Hedley C. A. Carr. 1999. "Circulating Tumor Cells After Surgery," *British Journal of Surgery* 86, no. 9: 1169–1176.

14 Steven L. Cohn. 1999. "Postoperative Immunosuppression and Its Role in Cancer Recurrence," *Cancer Chemotherapy and Pharmacology* 43, Suppl.: S1–S5.

15 Harold F. Dvorak. 2015. "Tumors: Wounds That Do Not Heal—Redux," *Cancer Immunology Research* 3, no. 1: 1–11.

16 Takuya Matsuda et al. 2020. "Inflammatory Response After Surgery and Its Impact on Cancer Progression," *International Journal of Clinical Oncology* 25, no. 2: 233–240.

17 Anecdotal patient testimony; see Clifton Leaf. 2013. *The Truth in Small Doses: Why We're Losing the War on Cancer—and How to Win It* (New York: Simon & Schuster).

18 Sean Byars, Stephen Stearns, and Jacobus Boomsma. 2018. "Childhood Surgery and Later Disease Risk," *JAMA Otolaryngology–Head & Neck Surgery* 144, no. 1: 27–34.

19 Sayer Ji. 2020. *Regenerate: Unlocking Your Body's Radical Resilience Through the New Biology* (New York: Hay House).

20 Lois B. Travis et al. 2010. "Testicular Cancer Survivorship: Research Strategies and Recommendations," *Journal of the National Cancer Institute* 102, no. 15: 1114–1130.

21 G. Morgan, R. Ward, and M. Barton. 2004. "The Contribution of Cytotoxic Chemotherapy to 5-Year Survival in Adult Malignancies," *Clinical Oncology* 16, no. 8: 549–560.

22 David J. Grignon and Paul E. Peters. 1996. "The Discovery of Chemotherapy from Mustard Gas," *Annals of Oncology* 7, no. 7: 719–724.

23 Alfred Gilman and Frederick S. Philips. 1946. "The Biological Actions and Therapeutic Applications of the β-Chloroethyl Amines and Sulfides," *Science* 103, no. 2686: 409–436.

24 R. F. Skipper et al. 1946. "Early Clinical Trials with Mustine in Lymphoma," *Cancer Research* 6, no. 12: 685–692.

25 Gilman and Philips, "Biological Actions," 409–436.

26 Bruce A. Chabner and Dan L. Longo. 2019. *Cancer Chemotherapy and Biotherapy: Principles and Practice*, 6th ed. (Philadelphia: Wolters Kluwer).

27 Morgan, Ward, and Barton, "Contribution of Cytotoxic Chemotherapy," 549–560.

28 American Cancer Society, "Radiation Therapy for Cancer," 2022, www.cancer.org.

29 Eric J. Hall and Amato J. Giaccia. 2012. *Radiobiology for the Radiologist*, 7th ed. (Philadelphia: Lippincott Williams & Wilkins).

30 Ajay K. Bhatia et al. 2021. "Radiation-Induced Immune Suppression: Mechanisms and Implications," *Frontiers in Immunology* 12: 563.

31 M. E. Lomax. 2016. "The Long-Term Effects of Radiation Exposure," *Mutation Research* 770: 1–6.

32 Robert J. Gillies et al. 2012. "Evolutionary Dynamics of Carcinogenesis and Resistance to Therapy," *Nature Reviews Cancer* 12: 487–493.

33 Peter J. Little. 2003. "Radiation-Induced Genomic Instability," *International Journal of Radiation Biology* 79, no. 7: 427–436.

34 American Cancer Society, *Cancer Facts & Figures* 2022.

35 Harold F. Dvorak. 2015. "Tumors: Wounds That Do Not Heal—Redux," *Cancer Immunology Research* 3, no. 1: 1–11.

36 Max Gerson. 1958. *A Cancer Therapy: Results of Fifty Cases and the Cure of Advanced Cancer by Diet Therapy* (Bonita, CA: Gerson Institute).

37 Mina J. Bissell et al. 2000. "Tissue Architecture: The Ultimate Regulator of Breast Epithelial Function?" *Current Opinion in Cell Biology* 12, no. 6: 677–685.

38 Angus Dalgleish. 2022. "Rapidly Progressing Cancers Following COVID-19 Vaccination," *BMJ* Rapid Response.

39 Andrew Kirsch et al. 2023. "The Role of Immune Dysregulation in COVID-19 and Its Connection to Cancer Progression," *Cancers* 15, no. 2: 231–248.

40 Dalgleish, "Rapidly Progressing Cancers."

41 Shashi Kant Singh et al. 2022. "SARS-CoV-2 Spike Protein Interactions and Their Implications for Autoimmunity and Cancer," *Frontiers in Immunology* 13: 1020001.

42 Muin J. Khoury et al. 2010. "Genetic Contribution to Cancer Risk," *JNCI Monographs* 2010, no. 40: 14–18.

43 Bruce McEwen. 1998. "Stress, Adaptation, and Disease," *Annals of the New York Academy of Sciences* 840: 33–44; Paolo Vineis and David Kriebel. 2006. "Causal Models in Epidemiology: Past Inheritance and Genetic Effects," *International Journal of Epidemiology* 35, no. 2: 437–442.

44 Ferdinand Ang et al. 2023. "Estimated Lifetime Gained with Cancer Screening Tests," *JAMA Internal Medicine* 183, no. 8: 902–912.

45 Ibid.; National Institutes of Health, "To Screen or Not to Screen? The Benefits and Harms of Screening Tests," *NIH News in Health*, March 2017.

46 Hyeong Sik Ahn, Hyun Jung Kim, and H. Gilbert Welch. 2014. "Korea's Thyroid-Cancer Epidemic—Screening and Overdiagnosis," *New England Journal of Medicine* 371, no. 19: 1765–1767.

47 Stacy Loeb and William J. Catalona. 2007. "PSA Screening for Prostate Cancer," *Urologic Oncology* 25, no. 6: 516–520.

48 Laura J. Esserman et al. 2014. "Addressing Overdiagnosis and Overtreatment in Cancer: A Prescription for Change," *The Lancet Oncology* 15, no. 6: e234–e242.

49 National Institute of Environmental Health Sciences, "Autoimmune Diseases," 2020, www.niehs.nih.gov/health/topics/autoimmune.

50 National Institute of Environmental Health Sciences, "Environmental Factors and Autoimmune Disease: What We Know and What We Don't," NIH, 2020.

51 Alessio Fasano. 2019. "Leaky Gut and Autoimmune Diseases: From Molecular Mechanisms to Clinical Applications," *Journal of Clinical Investigation* 129, no. 4: 1319–1331.

52 Lawrence Steinman. 2002. "Infection and Autoimmunity," *New England Journal of Medicine* 347, no. 12: 911–920.

53 G. Cooper et al. 2018. "Toxic Chemical Exposure and Autoimmunity," *Autoimmunity Reviews* 17, no. 9: 857–872.

54 Yehuda Shoenfeld and Nancy Agmon-Levin. 2011. "ASIA: Autoimmune/ Inflammatory Syndrome Induced by Adjuvants," *Journal of Autoimmunity* 36, no. 1: 4–8.

55 Yehuda Shoenfeld et al. 2020. "Vaccines and Autoimmunity: Considerations in Current Medicine," *Lupus* 27, no. 9: 1392–1398.

56 Andrea Janegová, Pavol Janega, Boris Rychlý, Kristína Kuracinová, and Pavel

Babal. 2015. "The Role of Epstein-Barr Virus Infection in the Development of Autoimmune Thyroid Diseases," *Endokrynologia Polska* 66 (2): 132–136.

57 Khalid M. Almutairi, Suliman A. Alghamdi, Ibrahim A. Aljuaid, Ali A. Alshehri, and Huda A. Alrubaian. 2023. "Exposure to Pesticides and the Risk of Hypothyroidism: A Systematic Review and Meta-analysis," *BMC Public Health* 23 (1): 1760; Marta Ziemińska, Ewelina Bilska, Joanna Kamińska, and Monika Czerska. 2025. "Toxic Heavy Metals and the Thyroid: An Updated Review," *PeerJ* 13: e18962.

58 Xiahe Publishing. 2023. "Gluten Is a Proinflammatory Inducer of Auto-immunity," *Journal of Translational Autoimmunity*.

Chapter 7

1 "How Does the Human Brain Work?" n.d. Caltech Science Exchange. https://scienceexchange.caltech.edu/topics/neuroscience/how-the-brain-works.

2 Irene Lyon n.d. "Traumatic Stress Physiology Has an Unpredictable Response," https://irenelyon.com/2018/06/11/traumatic-stress-physiology-has-an-unpredictable-response/.

3 Kendra Cherry 2024. "What Is the Fight-or-Flight Response?" Verywell Mind. https://www.verywellmind.com/what-is-the-fight-or-flight-response-2795194.

4 Bruce H. Lipton 2016. *The Biology of Belief 10th Anniversary Edition: Unleashing the Power of Consciousness, Matter & Miracles*. N.p.: HayHouse. https://www.brucelipton.com/product/the-biology-of-belief/.

5 Charles E. Herdendorf n.d. "Five States Take Steps to Halt Lake Erie Pollution." https://www.ebsco.com/research-starters/history/five-states-take-steps-halt-lake-erie-pollution.

6 Owen Stockdale et al. 2024. "Revitalizing Fields and Balance Sheets through Regenerative Farming." https://www.mckinsey.com/industries/agriculture/our-insights/revitalizing-fields-and-balance-sheets-through-regenerative-farming.

Chapter 8

1 Caroline Leaf. 2013. *Switch on Your Brain: The Key to Peak Happiness, Thinking, and Health* (Grand Rapids, MI: Baker Books).

2 Bruce H. Lipton. 2016. *The Biology of Belief: Unleashing the Power of Consciousness, Matter, and Miracles*, 10th Anniversary ed. (Hay House); Herbert Benson and Miriam Z. Klipper. 2000. *The Relaxation Response* (New York: HarperTorch).

3 Herbert Benson and Miriam Z. Klipper. 2000. *The Relaxation Response* (New York: HarperTorch); Shelley E. Taylor et al. 1990. "Psychological Resources, Positive Illusions, and Health," *American Psychologist* 45, no. 5: 513–531.

4 Glen Rein. 1996. "Effect of Conscious Intention on Human DNA," *Proceedings of the International Forum on New Science*: 338–348; Dean Ornish et al. 2008. "Changes in Prostate Gene Expression in Men Undergoing an Intensive Nutrition and Lifestyle Intervention," *Proceedings of the National Academy of Sciences* 105, no. 24: 8369–8374.

5   J. Bruce Moseley et al. 2002. "A Controlled Trial of Arthroscopic Surgery for Osteoarthritis of the Knee," *New England Journal of Medicine* 347, no. 2: 81–88.

6   Morton Prince. 1906. *The Dissociation of a Personality* (New York: Longmans, Green, and Co.); Richard P. Kluft. 1984. "Multiple Personality Disorder," *Psychiatric Clinics of North America* 7, no. 1: 9–29.

7   Donald A. McCaul. 1981. "The Nocebo Effect: Pain from Expectation," *Pavlovian Journal of Biological Science* 16, no. 3: 140–143; Luana Colloca and Fabrizio Benedetti. 2007. "Nocebo Hyperalgesia: How Anxiety Is Turned into Pain," *Current Opinion in Anaesthesiology* 20, no. 5: 435–439.

8   Shelley E. Taylor et al. 1990. "Psychological Resources, Positive Illusions, and Health," *American Psychologist* 45, no. 5: 513–531.

9   K. L. Kirschbaum et al. 2001. "Placebo Effects in Asthma: Subjective and Objective Outcomes," *New England Journal of Medicine* 345, no. 2: 103–107.

10 D. D. Price et al. 2008. "Placebo Analgesia: A Model for Understanding the Mechanisms of Placebo Effects," *Neuroscience* 9, no. 1: 339–353.

11 A. Kaptchuk et al. 2010. "Placebos without Deception: A Randomized Controlled Trial in Irritable Bowel Syndrome," *PLoS One* 5, no. 12: e15591; P. J. Whorwell et al. 1986. "Colitis Placebo Study," *Lancet* 1, no. 8482: 1232–1234.

12 J. Boivin et al. 1995. "Placebo Effect in Infertility Treatment," *Human Reproduction* 10, no. 12: 3251–3255.

13 Fabrizio Benedetti. 2008. "Mechanisms of Placebo and Placebo-Related Effects Across Diseases and Treatments," *Annual Review of Pharmacology and Toxicology* 48: 33–60.

14 Irving Kirsch et al. 2002. "The Emperor's New Drugs: An Analysis of Antidepressant Medication Data Submitted to the FDA," *Prevention & Treatment* 5, no. 1: 23; Joanna Moncrieff. 2007. "The Myth of the Chemical Cure: A Critique of Psychiatric Drug Treatment," *British Medical Journal* 335, no. 7611: 243–245.

15 Irving Kirsch. 2010. *The Emperor's New Drugs: Exploding the Antidepressant Myth* (New York: Basic Books).

16 Eric R. Kandel. 2001. "Neurobiology: Learning and Memory," *Science* 294, no. 5544: 1030–1038.

17 Jeffrey M. Schwartz and Sharon Begley. 2003. *The Mind and the Brain: Neuroplasticity and the Power of Mental Force* (New York: Harper Perennial).

18 Martin Seligman, 2006. *Learned Optimism: How to Change Your Mind and Your Life* (New York: Vintage Books).

19 Curt P. Richter. 1957. "On the Phenomenon of Sudden Death in Animals and Man," *Psychosomatic Medicine* 19, no. 3: 191–198; M. A. Matthews. 2011. "Hope and Survival: The Curt Richter Rat Experiment Revisited," *Journal of Behavioral Medicine* 34, no. 4: 319–330.

Chapter 9

1   Allan L. Adkin and Mark G. Carpenter. 2018. "Postural Threat and Anxiety: Inter-Relationships with Postural Control," *Neuroscience & Biobehavioral*

Reviews 94: 19–36; Karin Roelofs 2017. "Freeze for Action: Neurobiological Mechanisms in Animal and Human Freezing," *Philosophical Transactions of the Royal Society B: Biological Sciences* 372 (1718): 20160206.

2   Martin Picard, Bruce S. McEwen, and Carmen Sandi. 2018. "Mitochondrial Psychobiology: The Role of Mitochondria in Stress, Behavior, and Psychiatric Disorders," *Neuroscience and Biobehavioral Reviews* 84: 292–310; Douglas C. Wallace. 2012. "Mitochondria and Cancer," *Nature Reviews Cancer* 12, no. 10: 685–698.

3   Batya Swift Yasgur 2025. "While You Were Sleeping, the Brain's 'Waste Disposal System' Was at Work," *Medscape Medical News*, August 25, 2025. Accessed [August 29, 2025]; Jeffrey J. Iliff et al. 2012. "A Paravascular Pathway Facilitates CSF Flow Through the Brain Parenchyma and the Clearance of Interstitial Solutes, Including Amyloid β," *Science Translational Medicine* 4, no. 147: 147ra111; Lulu Xie et al. 2013. "Sleep Drives Metabolite Clearance from the Adult Brain," *Science* 342, no. 6156: 373–377.

4   SageMED. 2022. "The Benefits of Morning Sunlight for Your Health," *Sage Integrative Medicine*, June 30, 2022; CircadianBiology.com. n.d. "Light and the Circadian System," CircadianBiology.com. Accessed August 29, 2025.

5   Andrea Zaccaro et al. 2018. "How Breath-Control Can Change Your Life: A Systematic Review on Psycho-Physiological Correlates of Slow Breathing," *Frontiers in Human Neuroscience* 12: 353; Richard P. Brown and Patricia L. Gerberg. 2005. "Sudarshan Kriya Yogic Breathing in the Treatment of Stress, Anxiety, and Depression: Part II—Clinical Applications and Guidelines," *Journal of Alternative and Complementary Medicine* 11, no. 4: 711–717.

Chapter 10

1   Marion Nestle. 2013. *Food Politics: How the Food Industry Influences Nutrition and Health* (Berkeley: University of California Press); Michael Moss. 2013. *Salt Sugar Fat: How the Food Giants Hooked Us* (New York: Random House).

2   Bruce H. Lipton. 2016. *The Biology of Belief: Unleashing the Power of Consciousness, Matter, and Miracles*, 10th Anniversary ed. (Carlsbad, CA: Hay House).

3   Tim Spector. 2015. *The Diet Myth: Why the Secret to Health and Weight Loss Is Already in Your Gut* (New York: Abrams Press).

4   Ashley N. Gearhardt, William R. Corbin, and Kelly D. Brownell. 2009. "Food Addiction: An Examination of the Diagnostic Criteria for Dependence," *Journal of Addiction Medicine* 3, no. 1: 1–7.

5   Robert H. Lustig. 2012. *Fat Chance: Beating the Odds Against Sugar, Processed Food, Obesity, and Disease* (New York: Hudson Street Press).

6   Dariush Mozaffarian. 2016. "Dietary and Policy Priorities for Cardiovascular Disease, Diabetes, and Obesity," *Circulation* 133, no. 2: 187–225.

7   Nora D. Volkow et al. 2008. "Overlapping Neuronal Circuits in Addiction and Obesity: Evidence of Systems Pathology," *Philosophical Transactions of the Royal Society B* 363, no. 1507: 3191–3200.

8   Sayer Ji. 2020. *Regenerate: Unlocking Your Body's Radical Resilience through the New Biology* (New York: Hay House).

9   Jan Lotvall et al. 2014. "Extracellular Vesicles: Communication, Cargo and Function in Health and Disease," *Nature Reviews Molecular Cell Biology* 15, no. 12: 763–774.

10 Chen-Yu Zhang et al. 2012. "Exogenous Plant MIR168a Specifically Targets Mammalian LDLRAP1: Evidence of Cross-Kingdom Regulation by microRNA," *Cell Research* 22, no. 1: 107–126.

11 David R. Montgomery and Anne Biklé. 2022. *What Your Food Ate: How to Heal Our Land and Reclaim Our Health* (New York: W. W. Norton & Company); David R. Montgomery et al. 2022. "Soil Health and Nutrient Density: Preliminary Comparison of Regenerative and Conventional Farming," *PeerJ* 10): e12848.

12 Jordan Rubin. 2004. *The Maker's Diet* (Lake Mary, FL: Siloam Press).

13 Weston A. Price. 1939. *Nutrition and Physical Degeneration* (La Mesa, CA: Price-Pottenger Nutrition Foundation, 2008); Sally Fallon Morell. 2010. *Nourishing Traditions: The Cookbook That Challenges Politically Correct Nutrition and the Diet Dictocrats*, 2nd ed. (Washington, DC: NewTrends).

14 Nina Teicholz. 2014. *The Big Fat Surprise: Why Butter, Meat and Cheese Belong in a Healthy Diet* (New York: Simon & Schuster).

15 Fred A. Kummerow. 2015. "Dietary Trans Fats and Human Health," *Annals of the New York Academy of Sciences* 1357, no. 1: 1–20.

16 Valter D. Longo and Satchidananda Panda. 2016. "Fasting, Circadian Rhythms, and Time-Restricted Feeding in Healthy Lifespan," *Cell Metabolism* 23, no. 6: 1048–1059.

17 Noboru Mizushima and Masaaki Komatsu. 2011. "Autophagy: Renovation of Cells and Tissues," *Cell* 147, no. 4: 728–741.

18 Mindy Pelz. 2022. *Fast Like a Girl: A Woman's Guide to Using the Healing Power of Fasting to Burn Fat, Boost Energy, and Balance Hormones* (Carlsbad, CA: Hay House).

19 Iain H. Campbell et al. 2025. "Ketogenic Diet for Bipolar Disorder: Clinical Outcomes in a Proof-of-Concept Trial," *Frontiers in Psychiatry* 16: 1–12.

20 Matthew K. Taylor et al. 2022. "Ketogenic Diet in the Treatment of Mood and Psychotic Disorders," *Current Opinion in Psychiatry* 35, no. 5: 356–362.

21 Stanford Medicine, "Ketogenic Diet Improves Brain Metabolism in Severe Mental Illness: New Clinical Findings," *Stanford News*, March 2024.

22 Eric H. Kossoff et al. 2009. "Optimal Clinical Management of Children Receiving the Ketogenic Diet: Recommendations of the International Ketogenic Diet Study Group," *Epilepsia* 50, no. 2: 304–317.

23 Anu Sharma et al. 2022. "Ketogenic Diet Intervention in Patients with Type 2 Diabetes and Depression: A Pilot Trial," *Frontiers in Psychiatry* 13: 870–882.

24 Hai-Xia Wang et al. 2021. "Ketogenic Diet and Insulin Resistance: Insights into Mechanisms and Clinical Applications," *Signal Transduction and Targeted Therapy* 6: 92–104.

Chapter 11

1   U.S. Environmental Protection Agency. *Why Indoor Air Quality is Important in Schools.* https://www.epa.gov/iaq-schools/why-indoor-air-quality-important-schools.

2   Centers for Disease Control and Prevention (CDC). *Fourth National Report on Human Exposure to Environmental Chemicals, Updated Tables,* March 2021.

3   Environmental Working Group (EWG). *Body Burden: The Pollution in Newborns.* Washington, D.C.: EWG, 2005.

4   D.-H. Lee et al. 2023. "Association of Persistent Organic Pollutants with Disease Prevalence," *Environmental Research* 224.

5   Christopher Exley. 2017. "Aluminum in Brain Tissue in Familial Alzheimer's Disease," *Journal of Alzheimer's Disease* 55, no. 2: 897–906.

6   Dana Loomis et al. 2015. "Carcinogenicity of Benzene, Toluene and Xylene: Evaluation by the International Agency for Research on Cancer," *Cochrane Database of Systematic Reviews.* https://pmc.ncbi.nlm.nih.gov/articles/PMC5017538/.

7   Leah Schinasi and Maria E. Leon. 2014. "Non-Hodgkin Lymphoma and Occupational Exposure to Agricultural Pesticide Chemical Groups and Active Ingredients: A Systematic Review and Meta-Analysis," *International Journal of Environmental Research and Public Health* 11, no. 4: 4449–4527.

8   Shanna H. Swan et al. 2017. "Temporal Trends in Sperm Count: A Systematic Review and Meta-Regression Analysis," *Human Reproduction Update* 23, no. 6: 646–659.

9   Carmen Messerlian et al. 2016. "Urinary Phthalate Metabolites and Ovarian Reserve among Women Undergoing In Vitro Fertilization: Results from the EARTH Study," *Environmental Health Perspectives* 124, no. 6: 831–839; Russ Hauser et al. 2016. "Urinary Phthalate Metabolite Concentrations and Reproductive Outcomes among Women Undergoing In Vitro Fertilization: Results from the EARTH Study," *Environmental Health Perspectives* 124, no. 6: 831–839; Shelby J. Ferguson et al. 2011. "Urinary Bisphenol A Associations with Ovarian Response among Women Undergoing IVF," *Human Reproduction* 26, no. 10: 2613–2621; and Irene Souter et al. 2013. "Urinary Bisphenol A Concentrations and Implantation Failure among Women Undergoing In Vitro Fertilization," *Environmental Health Perspectives* 121, no. 4: 450–456.

10 S. J. Vagi et al. 2014. "Human Exposure to Hormone-Disrupting Chemicals and Their Effects on Reproductive Health," *Environmental Health Perspectives* 122, no. 9: 875–881. Chirag J. Patel et al. 2017. "Chronic Exposure and Epigenetic Impact of Endocrine Disrupting Chemicals: Transgenerational Evidence," *Toxicology Letters* 280: 174–183. G. N. Nassar et al. 2023. "Endocrine Disruptors: Mechanisms and Effects on Reproductive Health," *Frontiers in Endocrinology.* https://www.frontiersin.org/journals/endocrinology/articles/10.3389/fendo.2023.1324993/.

Chapter 12

1 Environmental Working Group (EWG). 2024. *Survey Finds Use of Personal Care Products Has Increased Since 2004— What That Means for Your Health.* Washington, DC: Environmental Working Group. https://www.ewg.org/research /survey-finds-use-personal-care-products-2004-what-means-your-health.

2 Russell L. Blaylock. 1997. "Excitotoxins in Foods," *Health and Nutrition Update* 8, no. 2: 1–6.

3 Environmental Defence. *Heavy Metal Hazard: The Health Risks of Hidden Heavy Metals in Face Makeup.* Toronto, 2011.

4 Environmental Working Group (EWG). *Skin Deep® Cosmetics Database.* Accessed 2024. https://www.ewg.org/skindeep/.

5 Anne Steinemann. 2016. "Fragranced Consumer Products: Exposures and Effects from Emissions," *Air Quality, Atmosphere & Health* 9, no. 8; Ki-Hyun Kim et al. 2022. "Volatile Organic Compounds and Their Roles in Neurotoxicity and Neurobehavioral Effects," *Environmental Research* 204: 112010; Ya-Nan Yuan et al. 2023. "Prenatal Exposure to Volatile Organic Compounds and Neurodevelopmental Outcomes in Children: A Systematic Review," *Environment International* 173: 107865.

6 Philippa D. Darbre. 2005. "Aluminium and the Human Breast," *Journal of Inorganic Biochemistry* 99, no. 9: 1912–1919.

7 National Toxicology Program (NTP). *Monograph on the Systematic Review of Fluoride Exposure and Neurodevelopmental and Cognitive Health Effects.* U.S. Department of Health and Human Services, 2023. https://ntp.niehs.nih.gov /research/assessments/noncancer/completed/fluoride.

8 William W. Nazaroff and Charles J. Weschler. 2004. "Cleaning Products and Air Fresheners: Exposure to Primary and Secondary Air Pollutants," *Atmospheric Environment* 38, no. 18: 2841–2865.

9 Erin M. R. Clayon, Kimberly J. Todd, and Rachel E. Bridge. 2011. "Exposure to Household Cleaning Products and Respiratory Health in Adults," *Occupational and Environmental Medicine* 68, no. 12: 914–919.

10 Environmental Working Group (EWG). *PFAS Contamination in the U.S.* Updated 2022. https://www.ewg.org/interactive-maps/pfas_contamination.

11 Robert Bilott. 2016. *Exposure: Poisoned Water, Corporate Greed, and One Lawyer's Twenty-Year Battle Against DuPont.* (New York: Atria Books).

12 Jeff D. Weidenhamer et al. 2017. "Metal Exposures from Aluminum Cookware: An Unrecognized Public Health Risk in Developing Countries," *Science of the Total Environment* 579: 805–813.

13 Johanna R. Rochester and Ashley L. Bolden. 2015. "Bisphenol S and F: A Systematic Review and Comparison of the Hormonal Activity of Bisphenol A Substitutes," *Environmental Health Perspectives* 123, no. 7: 643–650; G. González-Castro, M. Espinoza, E. Escalona-Segura, and A. Ramírez-Cahero. 2011. "Phthalates and Bisphenols Migration in Mexican Food Cans and Plastic Food Containers," *Bulletin of Environmental Contamination and Toxicology* 86, no. 6: 627–631.

14 C. M. Villanueva, Manolis Kogevinas, Sylvaine Cordier, et al. 2007. "Assessing Exposure and Health Consequences of Chemicals in Drinking Water: Emerging Challenges and Needs for New Tools," *Environmental Health Perspectives* 115, no. 10: 1479–1486.

15 Keith W. Brown and Douglas R. Bishop. 2007. "Shower Water Exposure and the Risks from Inhalation of VOCs," *Journal of Exposure Science & Environmental Epidemiology* 17, no. 4: 321–328.

16 R. Bashash M. A. Thomas, B. Hu, et al. 2017. "Prenatal Fluoride Exposure and Cognitive Outcomes in Children at 4 and 6–12 Years of Age in Mexico," *Environmental Health Perspectives* 125, no. 9: 097017; Philippe Grandjean et al. 2019. "Developmental Fluoride Neurotoxicity: A Systematic Review and Meta-Analysis," *Environmental Health Perspectives* 127, no. 6: 064501.

17 National Toxicology Program (NTP). 2024. *NTP Monograph on the State of the Science Concerning Fluoride Exposure and Neurodevelopment and Cognition: A Systematic Review*. Research Triangle Park, NC: National Toxicology Program. Monograph 08, August 21.

18 U.S. Environmental Protection Agency (EPA), "Indoor Air Quality," Report on the Environment, updated 2023, https://www.epa.gov/report-environment/indoor-air-quality. Ruthann A. Rudel, David E. Camann, John D. Spengler, Leo R. Korn, and Julia G. Brody. 2003. "Phthalates, Alkylphenols, Pesticides, Polybrominated Diphenyl Ethers, and Other Endocrine-Disrupting Compounds in Indoor Air and Dust," *Environmental Science & Technology* 37, no. 20: 4543–4553.

19 University of Washington Department of Environmental & Occupational Health Sciences. "Cleaner Air Means Better Health at Every Age." 2022. https://deohs.washington.edu/hsm-blog/every-age-cleaner-air-means-better-health.

20 International Agency for Research on Cancer (IARC). *IARC Monographs on the Evaluation of Carcinogenic Risks to Humans: Non-Ionizing Radiation, Part 2: Radiofrequency Electromagnetic Fields*. Vol. 102. Lyon: WHO/IARC, 2013.

21 Madhuri Sudan et al. 2010. "Prenatal and Postnatal Cell Phone Exposures and Headaches in Children," *Open Pediatric Medicine Journal* 4: 46–52; Maninder S. Setia et al. 2025. "Radiofrequency Electromagnetic Field Emissions and Neurodevelopmental Outcomes in Infants: A Prospective Cohort Study," *Cureus*, accessed November 10, 2025, https://www.cureus.com/articles/381425-radiofrequency-electromagnetic-field-emissions-and-neurodevelopmental-outcomes-in-infants-a-prospective-cohort-study/.

22 Odette Wilkens. Testimony to the National Call for Safe Technology, 2024.

Chapter 13

1 Taylor Carter. 2025. "ICA's Contemporary Definition of Vertebral Subluxation," *International Chiropractors Association*, April 11, 2025. Accessed August 29, 2025. https://www.chiropractic.org/definition-of-vertebral-subluxation/.

2 V. M. Frymann 1966. "Relation of Disturbances of Craniosacral Mechanisms to Symptomatology of the Newborn: Study of 1,250 Infants," *The Journal of the*

American Osteopathic Association 65, no. 10 (June): 1059–1075. https://pubmed
.ncbi.nlm.nih.gov/5178520/.

3   Godfrey Gutman, MD. 1987. "Blocked Atlantal Nerve Syndrome in Babies and
     Infants," *Manuelle Medizine*, 5–10.

4   Vishwathsen Karthikeyan et al. 2023. "Management of Perinatal Cervical Spine
     Injury Using Custom-Fabricated External Orthoses: Design Considerations,
     Narrative Literature Review, and Experience from the Hospital for Sick Children.
     Illustrative Cases," *Journal of Neurosurgery: Case Lessons*, (March). https://pmc
     .ncbi.nlm.nih.gov/articles/PMC10550666/.

5   Rachna Bahl, MD 2024. "Assisted Vaginal Birth in 21st Century: Current Practice
     and New Innovations," *American Journal of Obstetrics and Gynecology* 230, no.
     3 (March): S917–S931. https://www.ajog.org/article/S0002–9378(22)02583–2
     /fulltext.

6   G. Gutmann. 1987. "Kinematic Imbalance Due to Suboccipital Strain in
     Newborns," Manuelle *Medizin* 25, no. 1 (1987): 5–10; Viola M. Frymann 1966.
     "Relation of Disturbances of Craniosacral Mechanism to Symptomatology of
     the Newborn: Study of 1,250 Infants," *The Journal of the American Osteopathic
     Association* 65, no. 10: 1059–1075.

7   Heidi Haavik and Bernadette Murphy. 2012. "The Role of Spinal Manipulation
     in Addressing Disordered Sensorimotor Integration and Altered Motor Control,"
     Journal of Electromyography and Kinesiology 22, no. 5 (October): 768–776. https:
     //pubmed.ncbi.nlm.nih.gov/22483612/.

8   Heidi Haavik and Bernadette Murphy. 2011. "Subclinical Neck Pain and the
     Effects of Cervical Manipulation on Elbow Joint Position Sense," *Journal of
     Manipulative and Physiological Therapeutics* 34, no. 2 (February): 88–97. https:
     //pubmed.ncbi.nlm.nih.gov/21334540/.

9   A. R. Bandeira, L. M. A. Telles, V. Araldi, et al. 2021. "Heart Rate Variability in
     Patients with Low Back Pain," *Scandinavian Journal of Pain* 22, no. 3: 425–435;
     Carlos Fernández-Morales, Luis Espejo-Antúnez, Manuel Albornoz-Cabello,
     Ángel Rufino Yáñez-Álvarez, and María de los Ángeles Cardero-Durán. 2025.
     "Autonomic Balance Differences Through Heart Rate Variability Between
     Adults with and Without Chronic Low Back Pain," *Healthcare* 13, no. 5: 509;
     Christopher Kent. 2017. "Heart Rate Variability to Assess the Changes in
     Autonomic Nervous System Function Associated with Vertebral Subluxation,"
     Research & Reviews: Neuroscience 1, no. 3: 14–19, https://www.rroij.com/open
     -access/heart-rate-variability-to-assess-the-changes-in-autonomic-nervous
     -system-function-associated-with-vertebral-subluxation-.pdf.

10   Deed E. Harrison, Ibrahim M. J. Oakley, Stephanie S. Hauser, et al. 2016.
     "Decreased Vertebral Artery Hemodynamics in Patients with Loss of Cervical
     Lordosis," *Medical Science Monitor* 22: 495–500; Nicholas Moser, Silvano
     Mior, Michael D. Noseworthy, et al. 2019. "Effect of Cervical Manipulation on
     Vertebral Artery and Cerebral Hemodynamics in Patients with Chronic Neck
     Pain: A Crossover Randomized Controlled Trial," *BMJ Open* 9, no. 5: e025219.

11   See, for example, Jäger and Pfirrmann, "Systemic Inflammatory Markers in

Non-Specific Low Back Pain"; Zhang and Popovich, "Systemic Inflammation and Its Contribution to Chronic Neuropathology after Spinal Cord Injury"; Hotamisligil, "Inflammation, Metaflammation and Immunometabolic Disorders"; Rochlani et al., "Metabolic Syndrome"; Leng and Mucke, "Neuroinflammation and Neurodegeneration in Alzheimer's Disease"; and Walker, Ficek, and West, "Peripheral Inflammation and Risk of Dementia."

12   Oscar Sugar 1978. "Adverse Mechanical Tension in the Central Nervous System: An Analysis of Cause and Effect; Relief by Functional Neurosurgery," *JAMA* 240, no. 25 (December). https://jamanetwork.com/journals/jama /article-abstract/362912.

13   Fraser C. Henderson Sr. "Neurological and Spinal Manifestations of the Ehlers-Danlos Syndromes," *American Journal of Medical Genetics*. https://pubmed.ncbi .nlm.nih.gov/28220607/.

Chapter 14

1   Anna Christovich and Xin M. Luo. 2022. "Gut Microbiota, Leaky Gut, and Autoimmune Diseases," *Frontiers in Immunology* 13. (June). https://pmc .ncbi.nlm.nih.gov/articles/PMC9271567/. Diana Yasinskaya. 2025. "How a Damaged Gut Triggers Inflammation," *Medical News* (July). https://medical-news .org/how-a-damaged-gut-triggers-inflammation/98098/.

2   "Gut Microbiome." n.d. *Cleveland Clinic*. https://my.clevelandclinic.org/health /body/25201-gut-microbiome.

3   GemmaFabozzi et al. 2022. "Endocrine-Disrupting Chemicals, Gut Microbiota, and Human (In)Fertility—It Is Time to Consider the Triad," *Cells* 11, no. 21 (October). https://pmc.ncbi.nlm.nih.gov/articles/PMC9654651/. G. B. Rogers et al. 2016. "From Gut Dysbiosis to Altered Brain Function and Mental Illness: Mechanisms and Pathways," *Molecular Psychiatry* 21, no. 6 (April): 738–748. https://pmc.ncbi.nlm.nih.gov/articles/PMC4879184/.

4   Umea University. 2021. "Antibiotics Linked to Increased Risk of Colon Cancer," *Science Daily* (September). https://www.sciencedaily.com/releases/2021/09 /210901090057.htm.

5   Umea University. 2024. "Antibiotic Usage Can Damage the Protective Mucus Layer in the Gut," *Science Daily* (September). https://www.sciencedaily.com /releases/2024/09/240912135846.htm.

6   Debora Rondinella et al. n.d. "The Detrimental Impact of Ultra-Processed Foods on the Human Gut Microbiome and Gut Barrier," *Nutrients* 17 (5): 859. https://pmc.ncbi.nlm.nih.gov/articles/PMC11901572/.

7   "The Power of Healthy Fats for Brain Health." 2023. *Scientific Diet* (November). https://scientificdiet.org/2023/11/the-power-of-healthy-fats-for-brain-health/.

8   Peter C. Lehman et al. 2023. "Low-Dose Glyphosate Exposure Alters Gut Microbiota Composition and Modulates Gut Homeostasis," *Environmental Toxicology and Pharmacology* 100 (May). https://pmc.ncbi.nlm.nih.gov/articles /PMC10330715/.

9   Marianna Marino et al. 2021. "Pleiotropic Outcomes of Glyphosate Exposure: From Organ Damage to Effects on Inflammation, Cancer, Reproduction and Development," *International Journal of Molecular Sciences* 22, no. 22 (November). https://pmc.ncbi.nlm.nih.gov/articles/PMC8618927/.

10 Federica Giambò et al. 2021. "Influence of Toxic Metal Exposure on the Gut Microbiota (Review)," *World Academy of Sciences Journal* (February). https://www.spandidos-publications.com/10.3892/wasj.2021.90.

11 Marta Gea et al. 2022. "Assessment of Five Pesticides as Endocrine-Disrupting Chemicals: Effects on Estrogen Receptors and Aromatase," *International Journal of Environmental Research and Public Health* 19, no. 4 (February). https://pmc.ncbi.nlm.nih.gov/articles/PMC8871760/.

12 Alana Biggers 2023. "Do antibiotics harm healthy gut bacteria?" *Medical News Today* (November). https://www.medicalnewstoday.com/articles/do-antibiotics-harm-healthy-gut-bacteria#worst-types.

13 Ingvar Bjarnason et al. 2018. "Mechanisms of Damage to the Gastrointestinal Tract from Nonsteroidal Anti-Inflammatory Drugs," *Gastroenterology* 154, no. 3 (February). https://www.gastrojournal.org/article/S0016–5085(17)36666–0/fulltext.

14 "The Impact of Stress on Gut Health." 2024. *The Institute for Functional Medicine,* (October). https://www.ifm.org/articles/gut-stress-changes-gut-function.

15 Alex Schulz. 2023. "Leaky Gut and the Immune System," *Health & Science Magazine* (September). https://www.health-sciencemagazine.com/the-immune-system/leaky-gut-and-the-immune-system.

16 Sara Gottfried 2024. "Leaky Gut and Autoimmune Disorders," *Dr. Sara Gottfried MD* (August). https://www.saragottfriedmd.com/leaky-gut-and-autoimmune-disorders/.

17 Yumna El-Hakim et al. 2022. "Impact of Intestinal Disorders on Central and Peripheral Nervous System Diseases," *Neurobiology of Disease* 165 (April). https://www.sciencedirect.com/science/article/pii/S0969996122000183.

18 Amy Myers. 2025. "How to Fix Leaky Gut with Collagen," *Amy Myers MD* (June). https://www.amymyersmd.com/blogs/articles/how-to-fix-leaky-gut-with-collagen.

19 Dominic E. 2025. "Gut-Healing Properties of Bone Broth: Research Review." GutNow. https://www.gutnow.com/medical-treatments/gut-healing-properties-of-bone-broth-research-review/.

20 Kathryn Burge et al. 2019. "Curcumin and Intestinal Inflammatory Diseases: Molecular Mechanisms of Protection," *International Journal of Molecular Sciences* 20, no. 8 (April). https://pmc.ncbi.nlm.nih.gov/articles/PMC6514688/.

21 "Hypochlorhydria (Low Stomach Acid): Symptoms, Tests, Treatment." n.d. Cleveland Clinic. https://my.clevelandclinic.org/health/diseases/23392-hypochlorhydria.

22 Maya Shetty. 2024. "More than a Gut Feeling: How Your Microbiome Affects Your Mood," *Stanford Lifestyle Medicine* (April). https://longevity.stanford.edu/lifestyle/2024/04/08/more-than-a-gut-feeling-how-your-microbiome-affects-your-mood/.

23   Marie L. Johnson 2025. "8 Fermented Foods and Drinks to Boost Digestion and Health," *Healthline* (March). https://www.healthline.com/nutrition/8 -fermented-foods.

24   Jeremy Appleton 2018. "The Gut-Brain Axis: Influence of Microbiota on Mood and Mental Health," *Integrative Medicine: A Clinician's Journal* 17, no. 4 (August): 28–32. https://pmc.ncbi.nlm.nih.gov/articles/PMC6469458/.

25   Akash Kumar et al. 2023. "Gut Microbiota in Anxiety and Depression: Unveiling the Relationships and Management Options," *Pharmaceuticals* 16, no. 4 (April): 565. https://pmc.ncbi.nlm.nih.gov/articles/PMC10146621/.

26   "Leaky Brain Syndrome: Symptoms, Causes, and Solutions." n.d. Sane Solution. https://sanesolution.com/vitaae/leaky-brain-syndrome-symptoms-causes-and -solutions/.

27   Lena Michaelis et al. 2024. "Confounder or Confederate? The Interactions Between Drugs and the Gut Microbiome in Psychiatric and Neurological Diseases," *Biological Psychiatry* 95, no. 4 (February): 361–369. https://www.science direct.com/science/article/pii/S0006322323013586.

Chapter 17

1   M. Irwin, J. McClintick, C. Costlow, M. Fortner, J. White, and J. C. Gillin. 1996. "Partial Sleep Deprivation Reduces Natural Killer Cell Activity in Humans," *Psychosomatic Medicine* 58(6), 493–498. https://pubmed.ncbi.nlm .nih.gov/7871104/; https://www.ted.com/talks/matt_walker_sleep_is_your _superpower/transcript.

2   Tina Kold Jensen, Cecilia Ramlau-Hansen, Jonatan Bloch, Niels Jørgensen, Katharina Toft Guldbrandtsen, Aleksander Giwercman, Niels E. Skakkebæk, and Anders Juul. 2013. "Association of Sleep Disturbances with Reduced Semen Quality: A Cross-sectional Study Among 953 Healthy Young Danish Men," *American Journal of Epidemiology* 177, no. 10: 1027–1037; Matthew Walker "Sleep Is Your Superpower." *TED2019*, filmed April 2019. Video, 19:18.

3   S.-S. Yoo, Hu, P. T., Gujar, N., Jolesz, F. A., & Walker, M. P. 2007. "A Deficit in the Ability to Form New Human Memories without Sleep," *Nature Neuroscience* 10(3), 385–392.

4   C. S. Möller-Levet et al. 2013. "Effects of Insufficient Sleep on Circadian Rhythmicity and Gene Expression in Humans," *Proceedings of the National Academy of Sciences*.

5   Karine Spiegel, Rachel Leproult, and Eve Van Cauter. 2004. "Impact of Sleep Debt on Metabolic and Endocrine Function," *Annals of Internal Medicine* 141, no. 11: 846–850.

6   Karine Spiegel, Rachel Leproult, Esra Tasali, and Eve Van Cauter. 2004. "Sleep Curtailment in Healthy Young Men Is Associated with Decreased Leptin Levels, Elevated Ghrelin Levels, and Increased Hunger and Appetite," *Proceedings of the National Academy of Sciences of the United States of America* 101, no. 21: 18232–18237.

Chapter 20

1 Chiros Hub, "Heart Rate Variability—Chiros Hub," accessed August 30, 2025, summary of study involving 539 adults with one chiropractic adjustment and four-week follow-up showing sustained HRV improvements.

2 Heidi Haavik et al. 2024. "Neuroplastic Responses to Chiropractic Care: Broad Impacts on Pain, Mood, Sleep, and Quality of Life," *Brain Sciences* 14, no. 11: 1124.

3 Kelly Holt et al. 2019. "The Effects of a Single Session of Chiropractic Care on Strength, Cortical Drive, and Spinal Excitability in Stroke Patients," *Scientific Reports* 9, no. 1: 2673—reported a 64.2% average increase in plantar flexor muscle strength following a single chiropractic adjustment in chronic stroke patients.

4 D. M. Rothwell, S. J. Bondy, J. I. Williams. 2001. "Chiropractic Manipulation and Stroke: A Population-Based Case-Control Study," Stroke 32, no. 5 (May): 1054–1060. https://pubmed.ncbi.nlm.nih.gov/11340209/.

5 J. David Cassidy et al., 2008, "Risk of Vertebrobasilar Stroke and Chiropractic Care: Results of a Population-Based Case-Control and Case-Crossover Study," Spine 33 (February): S176–183. https://pubmed.ncbi.nlm.nih.gov/18204390/.

Chapter 21

1 Joana Araujo et al. 2019. "Prevalence of Optimal Metabolic Health in American Adults: National Health and Nutrition Examination Survey 2009–2016," *Metabolic Syndrome and Related Disorders* 17, no. 1.

2 D. Douchi et al. 2021. "Exosome-Mediated Transfer of Caveolin-1 Promotes Adipogenesis," *Biochimie Open*. PMC11104918.

3 T. Rönn et al. 2015. "DNA Methylation and Gene Expression in Human Adipose Tissue—Obesity and Weight Loss," *Epigenetics*. PMC4562340.

4 J. De Toro-Martín et al. 2022. "Obesity-Induced Gene Expression 'Memory' in Human Adipose Tissue Post-Weight Loss," *Diabetology & Metabolic Syndrome*. BMC DMSJ.

5 Brian Buntz. 2023. "Semaglutide and GLP-1: Effects on Lean Body Mass Still Unclear," *Drug Discovery Trends*, November 27, 2023, updated March 18, 2024—citing the STEP 1 and SUSTAIN 8 trials showing that 39–40 percent of weight lost on GLP-1 drugs was lean mass.

6 Jason Fung. 2016. *The Obesity Code: Unlocking the Secrets of Weight Loss* (Greenville, SC: Greystone Books).

7 RR Wolfe. 2006. "The Underappreciated Role of Muscle in Health and Disease." *Am J Clin Nutr*.

8 M. W. Hulver et al. "Skeletal Muscle Lipid Metabolism with Obesity." *Obesity*, 2003.

9 R. C. Laker et al. 2018. "A Mitochondria-Focused Model of Metabolic Flexibility," *Cell Metabolism*.

10 A. Paoli et al. 2012. "Ketogenic Diet and Carb Cycling Effects on Body Composition and Performance," *J Nutr Metab*.

Chapter 22
1 Vijay Pande et al. 2024. "Investing in Function Health," Andreessen Horowitz (a16z), June 25.